MARK LEIGH

IS IT IN YET?
THE BIG BOOK OF SEXUAL FAILURES

JB
JOHN BLAKE

Published by John Blake Publishing Ltd,
3 Bramber Court, 2 Bramber Road,
London W14 9PB, England

www.johnblakebooks.com

www.facebook.com/johnblakebooks
twitter.com/jblakebooks

This edition published in 2015

ISBN: 978 1 78418 688 3

All rights reserved. No part of this publication may be reproduced, stored in a retrieval system, or transmitted in any form or by any means, without the prior permission in writing of the publisher, nor be otherwise circulated in any form of binding or cover other than that in which it is published and without a similar condition including this condition being imposed on the subsequent purchaser.

British Library Cataloguing-in-Publication Data:

A catalogue record for this book is available from the British Library.

Design by www.envydesign.co.uk

Printed in Great Britain by CPI Group (UK) Ltd

1 3 5 7 9 10 8 6 4 2

© Text copyright Mark Leigh 2015

The right of Mark Leigh to be identified as the author of this work has been asserted by him in accordance with the Copyright, Designs and Patents Act 1988.

Papers used by John Blake Publishing are natural, recyclable products made from wood grown in sustainable forests. The manufacturing processes conform to the environmental regulations of the country of origin.

Every attempt has been made to contact the relevant copyright-holders, but some were unobtainable. We would be grateful if the appropriate people could contact us.

DEDICATION

To ....

I thought of you when I bought this book.

From ....

DISCLAIMER

All the incidents featured (even the really freaky ones and the ones that make you squirm) are presented in good faith, having been previously reported as fact and sourced from a wide variety of diverse publications, news services, hospital records and the Internet. If names, dates, locations or eventual consequences are absent, that is because none were provided in the original source material. In addition, it should be noted that many stories turn up in multiple sources but with slightly different facts. To this effect, the author and publishers cannot accept responsibility for any inaccuracies and apologise in advance for any inadvertent errors in reporting.

Look, at the end of the day it's not that important. It's not a book about something heavy like Gurdjieffian theory, the financial derivatives market or quantum physics; it's a book about sexual failures.

WARNING

While this book is designed to amuse and entertain, it should also act as a warning. Although some of the sexual acts reported in these incidents might seem tempting – alluring even – please do not try them at home. Particularly the ones involving vacuum cleaners.

ABOUT THE AUTHOR

Mark Leigh has considerable first-hand knowledge of sexual failure, which makes him exceptionally well qualified to write this book – a process that he claims has been a very cathartic experience.

When he's not involved in embarrassing bedroom incidents and the subsequent recriminations, repercussions and regrets, Mark has found the time to write or co-write over fifty humour and trivia books on subjects as diverse as celebrities, extra-terrestrials, swearing pets and chatting people up at funerals.

And while he's not writing books or apologies, Mark steals pens and photocopier paper from his job in marketing. For more details visit www.mark-leigh.com

CONTENTS

INTRODUCTION	XIII
ACCIDENTS WILL HAPPEN	1
WHATEVER TURNS YOU ON	13
GOING SOLO	31
AWKWARD MOMENTS	43
JUST PLAIN STUPID	55
BEASTLY BEHAVIOUR	69
CLOTHES MAKETH THE MAN	81
PLANES, TRAINS AND AUTOMOBILES	91
SERIOUS SHORTCOMINGS	105
TAKEN FOR A RIDE	111
MISCELLANEOUS	123
S&M	133
STUCK!	139

NOT TONIGHT, DARLING...	151
SEX LAWS	159
FOOD FUN AND GAMES	163
FOR THE THRILL OF IT	167
SEX FOR SALE	177
EXHIBITIONISTS	187
OUCH!	199
BE SATISFIED WITH WHAT GOD GAVE YOU	209
PLAYING AWAY	217
YOU'RE NICKED!	223
THAT'S JUST WRONG!	233
SAYINGS ABOUT SEX	249

INTRODUCTION

My name is Mark Leigh and I'm a sexual failure.

My reputation in the bedroom precedes me, which is why the publishers felt that, when it came to bad sex, I was the obvious Go-To Guy. When *Is It In Yet?* was commissioned, I felt a real sense of pride that my achievements (or rather, lack of them) haaeen recognised – not that I've been associated with most of the incidents here but because I can recognise a story about sexual failure when I see one. For the purposes of this book, sexual failure isn't just confined to non-performance in the bedroom; it's any act of a sexual nature that didn't quite go according to plan or where any consequences were ignored. However, even I – and my litany of bad experiences and subsequent apologetic texts – was not prepared for some of the incidents I unearthed.

Like the so-called Swiss Cheese Pervert who exposed himself with pieces of Swiss cheese wrapped around his penis, the man who had sex with a stuffed toy in a busy supermarket, the man who could only climax when hit in the face with a pie or the couple that decided to have sex on a train track… with inevitable results.

Now, you've probably spotted a pattern emerging here. Most of the incidents involve men acting alone. If there's an object to be inserted where it shouldn't, or if there's something irresponsibly dangerous to rub your groin against, you can guarantee a man did it.

Why? Is it due to a sense of boredom or a taste for adventure? There are men and women far better trained than me to make that judgement. My role is just to act as curator for these stories.

And there's the rub (sometimes quite literally): which stories to use and which to leave out.

After sifting through thousands of news reports, I decided that, to merit inclusion, the incidents should be bizarre and amusing and, therefore, entertaining. And that's when it came down to a question of taste.

Having someone die from a heart attack during sex isn't inherently funny. Having someone die from a heart attack and trapping his partner underneath them for four days is (well, I think it is). Then there's flashing. It's a criminal offence and can be quite traumatic to victims but, when a flasher falls out of a first-floor window after dropping his trousers and pants and saying, 'Who wants some of this?' it just has to go in.

One thing that did surprise me in my research was the sheer inventiveness some people went to in order to achieve sexual pleasure. And when I say inventiveness, I really mean reckless disregard of consequences.

INTRODUCTION

So sit back, kick off your shoes, cross your legs and get ready for some of the most deviant, dumb and, quite frankly, disturbing stories of bad sex.

It's enough to make you celibate.

Mark Leigh
Surrey, England 2015

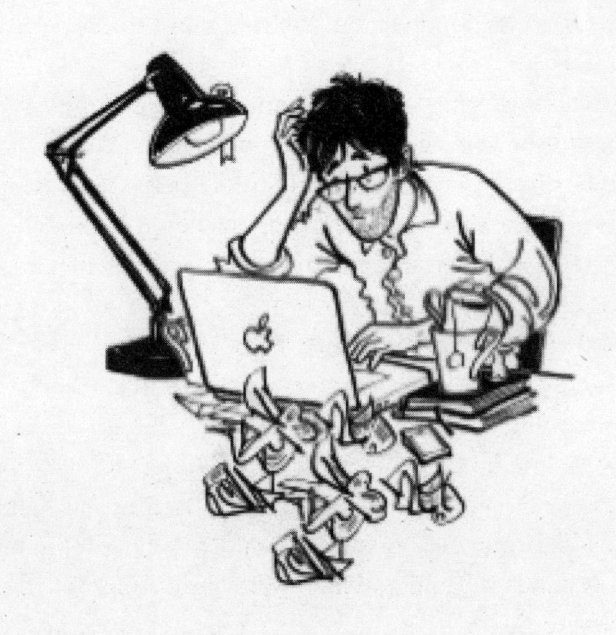

ACCIDENTS WILL HAPPEN

Whoever thought that a night of steamy passion would end with a couple being struck by lightning, someone being shot in the head or inadvertently super-gluing their own hand to their penis? As they say, even the best laid plans...

In 2013 a couple in the Chinese city of Wuhan decided to have sex against the glass window of their apartment. So energetic was the act that the window gave way, sending the couple to their death on the pavement below while still locked together.

A church official who presented himself to his local ER told staff on duty that his accident had occurred when we was hanging curtains at home. He decided to do this naked but, in the process, slipped off this ladder and fell right on to a potato...

Church organist Ian Kemp, forty-eight, from Teeside was found dead, naked, sealed in a large plastic bag with his legs bound at the shins by parcel tape and his wrists tied together with a silver chain. A vacuum cleaner had removed all the air from the bag. A spokesman for the Hardwick Baptist Church said Mr Kemp was a 'self-taught amateur', although it was not clear whether this comment referred to his organ playing or his apparent deviant tendencies.

Renowned American jazz trumpeter Jo 'Pootie' Newman was very fond of the ladies and, at the age of sixty-six, had surgery for a penile implant so he could maintain an erection. Unfortunately, the operation was unsuccessful and, on several occasions, a build-up of excess pressure caused the implant to explode and cause internal bleeding. One such incident occurred in a crowded restaurant. Mr Newman tragically died three years later from a blood clot on the brain.

In 2001 a man visited the emergency room of a small rural hospital in Ohio, presenting an injured penis. The doctor examining him saw that, although it wasn't bleeding, there was an 'appalling mid-shaft gash going at least halfway through.' The patient explained that he'd sustained the injury because he'd 'tried to make a horse do something she didn't want to do' and was bitten in the process.

A man presented himself to a Chicago hospital ER in July 2014 with his own hand super-glued to his penis: the result of a rather comical accident. It seems the patient was repairing a bedside lamp earlier that day and left the tube of glue next to it. That night he and his wife decided to have sex and he reached for what he thought was a tube of lubricant… you know what happened next.

Doctor Matthew Valente, who dealt with the case, commented, 'There wasn't just a small amount of glue. It wasn't just one finger. It was, in fact, his entire palm and all his fingers, which were tightly affixed to his genitals.'

Fortunately, the glue was dissolved with minimal damage to both hand and penis.

A man became suspicious that something was not quite right when he heard a vacuum cleaner running continuously in the trailer home next to his. On entering the premises, he found his fifty-seven-year-old male neighbour dead, naked and slumped over a vacuum cleaner, which had been fitted with a powered carpet-cleaning attachment. Rather than get his pleasure from the sucking power from the device,

IS IT IN YET?

the victim had been pressing his body against the motor. It was found that the areas of his body that had been in direct contact with the motor showed burn marks and that his testicles and buttocks had been tightly bound by a woman's tights. If that sight wasn't odd enough, the following items were found on the dining table: jars of lubricant, a glass of urine and a wooden table leg covered in faecal matter. It was determined that the victim had died from a heart attack.

General Sani Abacha was Nigeria's military head of state from 1993–98 who led one of the most brutal regimes the country had ever experienced. It was known that he had a number of concubines and, on the night of 8 June 1998, he commented to a few of his aides that he was 'in the mood for having a long sexual experience.' A number of women were brought to his room about midnight but, by the morning, Abacha was dead; thought to be a victim of that most deadly of combinations: a Viagra-fuelled orgy and a weak heart.

The body of Terrence Simmonds, a forty-nine-year-old from Oxford, was discovered in a home-made cocoon made of plastic bin liners. In what seemed to be a solo sex game, he'd used a vacuum cleaner to suck some of the air out of the bags but had failed to turn it off. After all the air had been drawn out, he'd suffocated.

ACCIDENTS WILL HAPPEN

A forensic journal titled 'Bizarre Impalement Fatalities: Where is the Implement?' published by the University of Münster, Germany included a case of a man who liked to insert one leg of an upturned wooden stool up his anus for sexual stimulation. One day he lost his balance and fell on to it, driving the leg all the way up to his diaphragm and rupturing his bladder and liver in the process. Before their examination, coroners were, at first, mystified as to the cause of death; there was no apparent murder weapon and there were no external injuries. Later it was discovered that, just before he died, the man had managed to remove himself from the furniture and his wife had hidden the stool.

A fifty-three-year-old Chinese man known only as Lu was found dead, naked in a chicken coop at his home. Police found the computer in his bedroom still playing porn and determined that, aroused by the porn, he went into the coop to masturbate. A combination of the cold temperature outside and his elevated heart rate from masturbation led to a fatal heart attack (the reason why he decided to masturbate in the chicken coop remains unknown).

A young man and his girlfriend were staying at his grandmother's and getting increasingly frustrated because they never had time alone. Eventually, the grandmother left the house to go shopping and the couple decided the time was right to have some fun. When looking for lubricant, they found the grandmother's nitroglycerin paste, prescribed for her angina, and decided it would do the job. It didn't. The paste caused their blood pressures to plummet and the grandmother returned to what was probably not the most treasured memory she has of the youngsters: unconscious and naked in her basement.

During sex, a New Zealand woman in her mid-forties was given a passionate love bite on her neck by her husband and found her left arm temporarily paralysed. Doctors found that the intense suction of the bite had caused bruising and a blood clot in an artery, which, in turn, had caused the woman to have a minor stroke.

An Australian woman was having very energetic sex in her hotel room when the vibrations from the bed rocking caused the ceiling light fitting to work loose and fall on her head, injuring her face and mouth. Instead of complaining to the hotel management, the woman tried, unsuccessfully, to sue her employers for physical and psychological damage. Her rationale was that the intercourse-related incident took place during a business trip.

ACCIDENTS WILL HAPPEN

In 2009 an unidentified Maryland couple were engaging in foreplay but the dildo they were using just wasn't stimulating enough. They decided they needed something a bit more vigorous, so their solution was to attach it to the blade of an electric saw, hoping the rapid in/out movement of the saw blade (and, therefore, the dildo) would have the desired effect.

You can guess what happened… The saw blade cut through the plastic dildo and the woman was rushed to hospital because of her injuries. Police decided not to press any charges, after concluding that the injury was a result of 'a consensual act between two parties and [that] no crime was committed.'

A nineteen-year-old cleaner was found dead and naked next to an electric floor polisher. While working, he'd been rubbing his naked groin against the machine to enjoy the vibrations. An inspection of the machine revealed that the polisher had been incorrectly earthed and that he'd been electrocuted.

An over-zealous man in China was kissing his girlfriend so vigorously that he reduced the air pressure in her mouth to such a degree that she ruptured her eardrum. A report in the *China Daily* gravely commented, 'While kissing is normally very safe, doctors advise people to proceed with caution.'

IS IT IN YET?

An unnamed young Indian woman eventually visited her doctor after suffering a serious cough, runny nose and fever for over six months. No medication seemed to help and, fearing something much more serious, the patient was sent for an X-ray. This revealed a condom stuck in one of her lungs. Apparently, she'd accidentally inhaled it while performing oral sex without actually realising.

Two Polish seventeen-year-olds, Beata and Kamil, were forbidden by their parents from marrying so, inspired by Romeo and Juliet, decided it would be better to live for eternity in death, rather than be separated in life. In April 1999 they went to a chemist to buy strong sleeping tablets but the pharmacist became suspicious and, instead, substituted these with laxative pills.

The couple booked into an economy room in a local hotel – a room without a toilet or bathroom – and took an overdose of what they assumed were the sleeping tablets before having passionate sex and then laying on the bed in each other's arms. It wasn't long before the laxative started to work. Having no toilet was one thing but the couple had no means to find another bathroom; as part of their plan, they had locked their room and thrown the key out of the window.

All they could do was scream for help; help that arrived too late.

The hotel manager had to fumigate the room afterwards and commented that the couple had found each other so disgusting afterwards that they called off their engagement.

ACCIDENTS WILL HAPPEN

A pre-med student and his date from the University of Arizona drove to a secluded spot on Mount Lemmon, overlooking the city of Tucson, to make out. They walked to an open knoll and, making a bed from their discarded clothes, started to have sex, failing to notice the heavy storm clouds and the low roll of thunder. Within moments, there was a blinding flash and a bolt of lightning found the highest point on the knoll – which happened to be the man's backside. The heat of the bolt melted his condom, fusing him and his girlfriend together. As if that wasn't bad enough, the man realised that, while he had survived the shock, albeit being in excruciating pain, his date hadn't – she lay dead beneath him.

This realisation caused him to vomit over her face but things then got worse. Attracted by the smell, a bear made his way over to the two lovers and began licking semi-digested food from the girl's face, before turning his attention to biting chunks from her face – just inches from the man's. Satisfied, the bear then moved off. The couple weren't discovered until the following morning, when a troop of hiking Girl Scouts came across them. Doctors called to the scene managed to separate the lovers. A hospital source was quoted as saying that, as a result of the lightning strike, the young man's penis resembled a 'small piece of cauliflower.'

Similar deaths have been reported where men have wrapped their penises in tin foil and then wired them to the mains. The result was not the ultimate orgasm they'd hoped for – just a painful death or, at best, permanent disfigurement.

IS IT IN YET?

An Illinois man, Bernie Carson, sued PT's Show Club for $200,000 for emotional distress, mental anguish and indignity, after being injured by a stripper during her performance. He had a front-row seat and claimed that the girl deliberately battered him around the head and neck with her massive breasts, which weighed an estimated 40 lbs each. The victim said that the experience had left him, 'bruised, confused, lacerated and sore.'

In a similar incident, in June 1998, Paul Shimkonis from Seminole, Florida sued the Diamond Dolls Club, claiming that being buffeted by stripper Tawny Peaks's (not her real name) massive sixty-nine-inch HH bosom, caused him whiplash during his bachelor party. He stated, 'The best way to describe it is like a concrete block hitting me in the forehead,' and sued the club for $15,000 of damages for 'bodily injury, disability, pain and suffering, disfigurement and mental anguish.' Rather than pursue conventional legal proceedings, Shimkonis had his case heard on the TV show *The People's Court*. He lost after the court heard that Ms Peaks's breasts weighed just 2 lbs each – well below the weight of concrete blocks.

A Louisiana couple discovered that sex and guns don't mix after one of them was shot in the head after an S&M session. It transpired that Rebecca Miller and Robert White had used the gun as part of their role-play but that Miller had accidentally shot her partner in the process. Local sheriff's-department spokesman Tony Mancuso described the incident as an 'accidental discharge of a firearm during consensual sexual activity.' Miller was later charged with negligent homicide.

Forty-year-old Jimmy 'The Beard' Ferrozzo was assistant manager of The Condor Topless Club in San Francisco and, after closing time one night in November 1983, he decided to frolic with one of the dancers – twenty-three-year-old Teresa Hill – on top of the club's grand piano. During their show of passion, a stray leg or arm accidentally knocked the button that raised the piano majestically into the air on a hydraulic lift – a popular gimmick used at the club. Ferrozzo died from asphyxiation when he was crushed between the piano and the ceiling, while the cushioning effects of his 220-lb body saved Hill, whose shouts the next morning alerted rescuers.

John Boyman, twenty-nine, of Erie, Pennsylvania, was visiting a local strip club, where he managed to get a table right at the front. He was having a good time, enjoying the antics of the club's star performer, Cherri Blossom. She removed her bra but, to Mr Boyman's disappointment, was wearing two small sequinned tassels over her nipples. Feeling short-changed, to Miss Blossom's and everyone else's surprise, he jumped on stage and attempted to remove the tassels with his teeth. His attempt on the first one was successful but, in his haste and excitement to remove the second, he swallowed it and choked to death.

A woman in Long Branch, New Jersey was hospitalised after performing a striptease for her boyfriend while seductively holding a shotgun. In the process, she accidentally shot one of her breasts.

In 2007 the naked bodies of two twenty-one-year-olds – Chelsea Tumbleston and Brent Tyler from Columbia, South Carolina – were found in the street early one morning by a passing cabbie. A police spokesman said, 'The driver was stunned. It's rather unusual to find two dead, naked people in the middle of the road.' He said the deaths were being treated as a tragic accident, adding, 'We believe they rolled off a roof while in the heat of passion.'

In an attempt to inject some excitement into her love-life, a German housewife decided to undress and then hide in the bedroom wardrobe, where she could surprise her husband. He was so surprised, in fact, that, when she jumped out of the wardrobe, he fell backwards through the bedroom door and stumbled down the hallway before falling backwards out of a window. He sustained serious but not life-threatening injuries.

WHATEVER TURNS YOU ON

Breasts, legs, hairy chests, bottoms even toes… the conventional 'turn ons' are well documented but what's far less well-known are actions that can also cause the same level of sexual arousal. Here, we're talking about incidents where people have got off by crushing insects, painting toenails, vomiting, watching others sneeze and throwing lard…

In July 2001 thirty-eight-year-old Richard Lee Sanders of Burnsville, Minnesota was charged with disorderly conduct after he approached three women on the street, complimented them on their fingernails and then, when the women proudly displayed their hands, grabbed them and began sucking on their fingers. The prosecuting attorney said that this was 'his weirdest case in sixteen years on the job.'

IS IT IN YET?

A survey conducted by Wisconsin researchers into the reason for nose-picking found that 0.4 per cent of those surveyed did it for sexual stimulation.

Toe-sucking is a well-documented fetish that's even practised by the criminal fraternity. In 1994 Italian police tried, unsuccessfully, to arrest a robber who would hold up shops in Pisa and then, before he left, force the female sales assistants to let him suck their toes.

'Crushing' is the sexual fetish whereby people become aroused by the sight of women's feet smashing small creatures like insects, fish and mice. Between 1998 and 2000, statutes in the US were enacted to target the practice and those posting Internet videos of animal cruelty were tracked down and arrested, forcing the online crush scene underground.

Ibrahim Gadzhiyev, thirty-five, of the Chechen Republic, was heavily into vampire sex, attacking and killing Lena Karaseva, a Miss Russia finalist, in 1996 before drinking her blood. After his arrest, the ex-mercenary confessed to thirteen other horrific murders and told detectives, 'I am a vampire. I attack people because I want to suck warm blood.' He told police he had sex with Lena while sinking his teeth into her neck and sucking her blood.

A detective commented, 'He cannot be human. He is like something out of a horror story.' The officer added that, when police asked Gadzhiyev to drink a litre of cow's blood to prove his twisted craving, he gulped it down in one go.

A man in Tifton, Georgia was apprehended after a car chase and convicted of public indecency after a series of incidents in which he would drive around in the nude, throwing chunks of lard at female victims.

It's not often that the words 'aroused' and 'vomit' are used in the same sentence but emetophilia is the condition of being sexually aroused when vomiting, being vomited on or watching someone vomit. Stefan Luckham claimed he suffered from that condition when he was arrested in 2007. He'd made women drink drain cleaner so he could become sexually aroused when they were violently sick.

Enough people are turned on by sneezing (either sneezing themselves or seeing someone else sneeze) that there's a very active sneeze-fetish forum. A typical discussion concerns people posting about sneezes they've heard. For example,

IS IT IN YET?

one member described a co-worker who has the 'cutest sneeze ever. She gives a big "Ahhhh", then makes the squeak sound of a pinched stifle, and then lets out a loud "Chooo".'

Responses to this sort of posting are both congratulatory and envious. One poster wrote, 'What I wouldn't do to work in a desk beside her.' Another said, 'That's great! I wish I could make a certain someone allergic to me.'

District Judge Andrew Duvall was a longstanding and upright member of the community of Bedford, Pennsylvania – until a twenty-one-year-old man appeared before him in 2001 on charges of public drunkenness and disorderly conduct. The judge offered the defendant a lighter sentence if he agreed to one thing… to let the judge shampoo his hair. Furthermore, he would reduce the sentence further if he could wash the hair of two of the accused's friends. The man agreed but the two friends he brought back were state troopers. The judge admitted his hair-washing fetish and resigned from office.

Most people know about necrophilia (getting turned on by dead bodies) or coprophilia (being aroused by faeces) but there are some equally bizarre (and disturbing) fetishes…
- Clowns (coulrophilia)
- Trees (dendrophilia)
- Burglary (harpaxophilia)
- Having insects crawl over your genitals (formicophilia)

WHATEVER TURNS YOU ON

- Sucking on someone's nose (nasolingus)
- Armpit hair (hirsutophilia)
- Fog (nebulophilia)
- Sacred objects (hierophilia)
- Stuttering (psellismophilia)
- The deformed (teratophilia)
- Tears (dacryphilia)
- Falling downstairs (climacophilia)
- Hair (trichophilia)
- Alien creatures (exophilia)
- Stone or gravel (lithophilia)
- Old people (gerontophilia)
- Pinching (thlipsosis)
- Stabbing or piercing the skin of someone (piquerism)
- Electric shocks (electrophilia)
- Mucus (mucophilia)
- Amputees (acrotomophilia)
- Using your partner like a piece of furniture (forniphilia)
- Statues or mannequins (agalmatophilia)
- Teddy bears (ursusagalmatophilia)
- Smells (ozolagnia)
- Catheters (catheterophilia)
- Shoes (retifism)
- Mucus (mucophilia)
- Using food for sexual pleasures (sitophilia)
- Pulling out your sexual organs by the roots (enderacinism)
- Licking eyeballs (oculolinctus)
- Scratching and itching (acarophilia)
- Enemas (klismaphilia)
- Strong and muscular women (sthenolagnia)

IS IT IN YET?

- Vomiting or being vomited on (emetophilia)
- Being eaten alive or eating someone else (vorarephilia)

An open verdict was recorded after a man's body was found on his bed, having been strangled by a shoelace. At the inquest, the coroner stated that the death could be explained by one of three things: murder, suicide or misadventure during a deviant sexual practice. The victim was found surrounded by cuddly toys, holding a wooden spoon in one hand.

A Tokyo mugger had a strange MO… he'd threaten people and make them hand over their contact lenses. After he was arrested, police discovered his fetish. His home contained 154 pairs of contact lenses and glasses.

Thousands of people die each year from autoerotic asphyxiation: the act of masturbating while robbing the brain of oxygen to create a feeling of ecstatic euphoria. Those seeking this 'high' may strangle themselves with cords, ropes, scarves or ties, or suffocate themselves by sealing their heads in plastic bags – but deaths occur when they go too far and fail to stop the asphyxiation. Two of the highest-profile victims have been INXS singer Michael Hutchence and actor David Carradine.

WHATEVER TURNS YOU ON

Closer to home, one of the best-known reports concerned Conservative MP for Eastleigh Stephen Milligan, who is believed to have died while pleasuring himself during a 'solo-bondage and self-strangulation sex act.' News reports state that, in 1994, his housekeeper found his body at his Chiswick home tied to a kitchen chair, naked apart from stockings and suspenders, with a plastic bag over his head and an orange in his mouth (although some reports say it was actually a satsuma).

The Trobiand islanders – part of the nation of Papua New Guinea – practise something called *mitakuku*, whereby, during lovemaking, they bite off their partner's eyebrows at the moment of climax.

A Tokyo newspaper reported the story of a local resident who had a huge fetish for women's socks; so much so, in fact, that, when he saw a woman in the street wearing socks inappropriately – i.e. down around her ankles – he assaulted her by rubbing spit in her hair.

The Associated Press reported the story of a New Jersey man who robbed twelve urologists' offices in revenge for them refusing to give him a prostate examination. The court heard that the man didn't need the procedure but just got pleasure from having the inspection.

A mugger, who was later caught by New York police, admitted stealing glasses from people in the street because he'd get sexually aroused wearing them in bed.

The American Journal of Forensic Medicine & Pathology reported the bizarre case of a sixty-year-old man found dead in his apartment, wrapped in fourteen different blankets with a plastic bag full of semen attached to his penis. Investigators discovered that the blankets had been taped to him and postulated that he'd laid them out with double-sided tape attached and had rolled into them, one by one, until he was cocooned in the middle, as a way to get his sexual thrills. Unfortunately, he'd suffocated in the process.

A man named only as S.L., from Arizona, revealed in a letter to *Forum* magazine that he could only make love to a woman if she had a limp. 'Not amputees or any weird stuff,' he explained. 'They just have to be slightly lame.' He went on to explain that he was in love with a girl who'd sprained her ankle playing tennis but that, after she recovered, he couldn't get an erection. Even putting on a limp for him had no effect.

WHATEVER TURNS YOU ON

Four women reported that a man had fondled and, in some cases, sucked their hair, while they were watching *Sleepless in Seattle* in a movie theatre in Grosse Point Woods, Michigan. All they could tell police was that he looked like Kenny Rogers.

Sex therapist Dr Robert Chartham reported on a man who would only make love to his wife if his feet were submerged in cold water. Their usual position for sex was with him sitting on the edge of the bath with his feet in the water and his wife facing him, straddling his lap.

A Los Angeles man known only by his nickname of Leonardo da Toenail was caught in 1981 after a number of complaints from young women at the University of Southern California. Leonardo had a very odd modus operandi and would target only those wearing open-toed footwear. Posing as a student, he would go into the university's library and sit opposite his target, take his books out and begin studying. He would then pretend to drop a pen and, while reaching under the table to pick it up, would surreptitiously paint the nail on the girl's big toe. If she didn't realise, he'd drop something else on the floor and paint the other one. When arrested, police found he was carrying sixteen bottles of nail varnish. However, he wasn't charged with any offence, since his victims felt foolish testifying against him.

IS IT IN YET?

Keith Everett, twenty-nine, went by the nickname of Jack the Crimper after his bizarre habit of creeping up on unsuspecting women and shampooing their hair for as long as he could before running off. In 1985 he was jailed for washing the hair of ten women in this way.

Thirty-three-year-old Jerome Wright of New York had a fetish about women's bottoms. Nothing too unusual about that, you may think, until you realise that the way he got his kicks was by firing a blow dart at them. He confessed to targeting the buttocks of at least fifty-five well-dressed women at the city's Pennsylvania station in the summer of 1990, firing a large pin at them through a drinking straw. He explained to police that fat women were his favourite targets, as their butts were easier to hit.

Someone else with an odd bottom fetish was thirty-two-year-old Terence Goodhew of London, who would creep up on girls waiting at bus stops in West Ham and try and set fire to their bottoms. When arrested in 1982, he refuted the police allegations and just told them, 'I'm careless with matches.'

Loli-can – or The Lolita Complex – is the name for the Japanese fetish that began in 1993, where men happily paid up to $60 for a pair of vacuum-packed used panties that once belonged to a schoolgirl, accompanied by a photo of her wearing them. Eager to cash in on this craze, one enterprising company even offered panties via street-vending machines in Tokyo.

A year later, the obsession had moved on and the craze was for schoolgirl saliva offered in a 50-ml bottle. Freshness was guaranteed; the saliva was refrigerated and certified as not being more than seven days old.

The Roman Emperor Domitian got his sexual kicks by slowly plucking out the pubic hair of his lovers, one by one.

Michael Kenyon, otherwise known as 'the enema bandit', unleashed a reign of terror on the residents of Urbana, Illinois at intervals between 1966 and 1975. Described as an 'obsessive enema lover', Kenyon would break into homes and administer enemas to his victims under gunpoint but was eventually arrested in connection with a number of armed robberies in suburban Chicago. It was during questioning that officers became aware that he was the enema bandit. He served six years in prison and was paroled in 1981 and was immortalised by Frank Zappa in his song 'Illinois Enema Bandit', recorded live in December 1976.

IS IT IN YET?

A policeman was jailed for six months for replacing a loo roll in his next-door neighbour's house with one that deviously contained a miniature camera, allowing him to view images on his TV of her on the toilet. The victim told the court, 'I knew something was up, as I usually use peach toilet paper.'

A man from Ohio had a very peculiar way of arousing himself; he'd play with himself until he achieved an erection and, at the moment of climax, would shoot himself with a gun. He wasn't entirely crazy though... he did wear a bulletproof vest.

Police in Ohio were called to a house when a man discovered his father lying face down on the couch, naked and not breathing. Medics on the scene pronounced the man dead but, when his body was removed, they discovered two unusual sights: burn marks around his genitals and a hole in one of the cushions in the position of his groin. On removing the cushion, they found two electric sanders fixed to the couch frame.

It turned out that the man had had a habit of putting his penis down the hole and enjoying the good vibrations of the sanders (with the sanding paper removed, of course). His death was caused by his orgasm shorting out one of the sanders, resulting in his electrocution.

WHATEVER TURNS YOU ON

In July 2009 Aberdeen police found Amy Henderson vigorously masturbating near a number of burning dustbins outside a McDonalds in the city's main shopping centre. Further investigations found petrol, rags and a lighter in her handbag. She later admitted starting the blazes because she suffered from pyrophilia – a sexual disorder that meant she was turned on by fire.

In a similar case, in 1997, two San Diego residents were charged with setting fire to various motor vehicles. They told the court that they did it for their twenty-seven-year-old friend Tammy Jo Garcia, who was aroused by the sight of burning cars.

Emperor Tiberius used to skinny dip in a pool filled with young boys, who would nibble on his penis as he swam.

In 2007 Canadian police were keen to track down an unknown masochist, who approached women and pestered them to kick him in the groin. While not a crime in itself, the police were worried that women might be in danger from his ulterior motives.

Women in northern Siberia are reported to show their interest in men by throwing slugs at them.

IS IT IN YET?

In 1994 thirty-three-year-old French art lover Michel Renet staged a twelve-day hunger strike to protest against a judge's refusal to permit him to legally marry the Venus de Milo statue.

Kevin Kirkland, a forty-four-year-old computer engineer from Shropshire, was found naked apart from his socks and boots, handcuffed to a tree in August 2010, with a cord also wrapped around his penis. The inquest into his death heard he had died from a combination of hypothermia and blood loss from cuts on his wrists, which were caused by his desperate attempts to escape, presumably after changing his mind.

Summing up on one of her cases, judge Anne Tyler commented that the man who appeared in her Ohio courtroom had 'what can only be described as a urine fetish.' He was arrested for collecting urine from male restrooms with the intention of drinking it.

In January 2012 thirty-four-year-old Christopher Bjerkness of Duluth, Minnesota was sentenced to four years of supervised probation for breaking into school gyms, sports complexes and rehabilitation centres and slashing rubber

WHATEVER TURNS YOU ON

exercise balls with a knife to fulfil a sexual urge. Bjerkness admitted that he can't explain his fetish but said he isn't a threat to people; only balls.

A fifty-one-year-old British man who practised auto asphyxiation was discovered dead, hanging from a tree. Police who searched his house found the following items: handcuffs, leg irons, a penis vice, scrotum weights, various electric-shock devices, a mace with chain and spiked ball, canes, whips and 107 pairs of leather gloves, of which twenty-nine were determined to have semen stains inside.

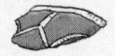

Author James Joyce admitted to being turned on by his lover's unwashed underwear.

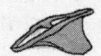

Over a long period of time, twenty-five-year-old Frank Ranieri from Staten Island, New York impersonated a police officer to win the trust of teenagers. He'd pay them $500 a time to let him stab them in the buttocks with a pin or a biro. One girl earned almost $6,000 in total and told the (real) police that she went along with it as she needed the money. Another recruited two of her friends, telling them, 'If you want to make some cash, he'll pay you a lot. It's not so bad.' Ranieri was arrested in June 2007 and charged with second-degree assault as part of a sexually motivated crime.

History doesn't record who suddenly thought, 'I want to increase my sexual performance, so I'll eat ambergris,' (a waxy substance found in the intestines of sperm whales) but the concept of the aphrodisiac exists in almost every culture.

It's easy to understand the origin of some aphrodisiacs. Foods that mimic certain body parts were supposed to aid those same body parts, which is why powdered rhino horn or the sea cucumber are notable aphrodisiacs in Asia.

Other aphrodisiacs are actually toxins that can enhance arousal. These include Spanish fly – an acidic beetle secretion that can cause a severe fever – and also fugu – or blowfish – which can lead to pleasurable tingling if it's prepared properly… or a painful death if it's not.

The following items, as bizarre as they sound, are all reported to enhance sexual performance.
- Cobra blood
- Powdered frogs' bones
- Tiger penis
- The milk of an ass combined with the blood of a bat
- Powdered cow dung dissolved in water
- Sheep's eyelids soaked in hot tea
- Pigeon excrement
- Live monkey brains
- Lizards soaked in urine
- Bull penis-and-testicle soup

WHATEVER TURNS YOU ON

- Menstrual blood
- Dolphin testicles
- Duck eggs containing a partially developed foetus
- Skink (lizard) flesh
- Wolf meat
- Rhino horn
- Leaf-cutter ants
- Dolphin testicles
- Bamboo urine
- Sea Cucumber
- Caterpillar fungus (a parasite than infects the brains of
- caterpillar larvae)
- Toad excrement
- Pigeon dung
- Melted fat from a camel hump
- Ambergris (intestinal secretions of the sperm whale)
- Blood from a dog that has eaten a crow that has eaten a
- centipede

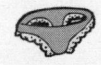

GOING SOLO

There's nothing wrong with masturbation, providing it's done in the comfort and privacy of your own home and not, as some of these incidents took place, in a public library, on a golf course, in a police van, a supermarket or the public gallery of a magistrates' court...

In March 1993 an elementary-school teacher and three other men were spotted on a golf-course fairway in North Little Rock, Arkansas, holding something other than golf clubs. They stood in a circle, masturbating and didn't even stop when approached by a police officer. He let them continue while he went to get back-up and, when he returned later with his partner to make the arrest, they were still doing it.

IS IT IN YET?

In April 2004 Toronto Police officers received a call about a suspicious incident at Agincourt Library. They found a man sitting in front of his laptop, masturbating with one hand and holding a cucumber with the other. The man – Fredrick Tennyson Davis, forty-nine – was charged with an indecent act. Constable David Hopkinson commented, 'He was not using the cucumber to pleasure himself, as far as I'm aware. It was held in his other hand – multi-tasking.' Hopkinson also added that he doubted whether David posed any danger to the library's staff or patrons, saying, 'I don't think he had any free hands to make any threat.'

In March 2008 a Polish building contractor was caught by a security guard in an intimate moment with a Henry vacuum cleaner in the Great Ormond Street Hospital staff canteen. The guard is reported to have told the man to 'clean himself and the hoover,' before asking him to leave, then reporting the incident. When later questioned by his employers, the contractor said that vacuuming in his underpants was 'a common practice in Poland.' He has since been fired.

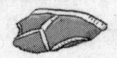

In July 2014 nineteen-year-old Parvinder Aullakh was charged with outraging public decency after being seen masturbating in a public place. The place he chose, however, wasn't the most discreet of places, being frequented by police and members of the legal profession: the public gallery at

GOING SOLO

Hammersmith Magistrates Court in West London. A court official stated that 'the teenager was escorted from court by police but continued with his actions.' He was sentenced on 7 April 2015.

Derek Bennett, twenty-six, was arrested in June 2014 after shoppers in an Oklahoma branch of Walmart reported him to be masturbating. Two customers saw him nonchalantly strolling up and down aisles with his penis out and reported him to security. Bennett ran out when police arrived but was soon caught. According to a local TV station, he immediately admitted to exposing himself, but said he was genuinely surprised he'd been spotted.

During a routine check-up in November 1991, Dr d'Avis of Illinois asked his patient for consent to check for haemorrhoids. The patient agreed but, during the rectal examination, the patient happened to glance round to see the doctor performing the examination with one hand and masturbating with the other. The case went to court and Dr d'Avis was convicted of assault and put on one year's probation.

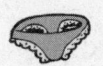

IS IT IN YET?

A thirty-four-year-old primary-school teacher was convicted in September 2007 following an incident in Clydebank, Scotland. He'd parked outside a local high school and was seen leering at students. What made his actions worse was the fact that, at the same time, he was observed pleasuring himself with an electric vibrator plugged into his car's cigarette lighter.

When Charles Veltman was arrested for possession of tools for the commission of a crime, police also found that he was carrying a home-made vibrator. Veltman admitted that he had planned to rob an electrical store because he'd run out of batteries.

Alone in her parents' Jacuzzi on a day in September 1999, Gemma Humphries was curious to see if she could arouse herself by directing the air jets towards her lady parts. Her search for a thrill left her in hospital with acute abdominal pain from air trapped in her abdomen – and the embarrassment of explaining how she suffered this injury.

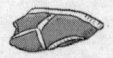

Polish housewife Joanna Kozlowska felt really horny and, with no vibrator to satisfy herself, improvised with a hand-held food mixer, using the vibrations to bring her to orgasm.

GOING SOLO

All would have been well had she not decided to use the makeshift sex aid in the bath. Joanna didn't die from the shock but it was strong enough to send her to hospital. She later blamed her husband for the accident, saying it was his fault for not tending to her needs.

A man from Lund in southern Sweden was arrested for masturbating in a public place. An obvious creature of habit, to the horror of the officers escorting him, he started masturbating again in the police van on the forty-minute drive to the police station.

The warden of a Mexican jail, Raul Díaz, got his kicks by masturbating while spying on prisoners enjoying conjugal visits. He did this over a long period undetected, until the time when he tripped on a roof skylight and fell through the roof on to a couple in the throes of passion. *La Cronica* newspaper reported that the warden died after hitting the concrete floor – and that a pair of binoculars and a pornographic magazine were found on his body.

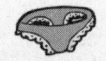

Masturbation is still outlawed in French Guiana. The law notes that this physical act 'is recognised as a common cause of insanity'.

IS IT IN YET?

A thirty-five-year-old man complaining of a pain in his bladder was found to have three small squirrel vertebrae in there. It was later discovered that the patient had practiced urethral masturbation using the bones of a squirrel tail. Poking objects into your penis for sexual stimulation is not that unusual and there are medical reports of other odd objects being removed from men's bladders: a long wax taper, needles, hairpins, plant stems and a sprig of wheat, to name but a few.

Nicola Paginton – a seemingly healthy thirty-year-old children's nanny from Cirencester – was found dead in her bed in July 2010 after she missed a few days at work and her employer and a friend broke into her home to search for her. According to newspaper reports, she was found semi-naked, with a vibrator by her side and a porn film playing on her laptop. The pathologist stated that the cause of death – a heart attack – was 'probably brought on by her state of arousal.'

An American woman who was starting her own business was working sixteen-hour days and had no time for any male company, let alone a boyfriend. Instead, she relied on a mains-powered vibrator for sexual stimulation. One night she fell asleep with the sex aid still running inside her, the motor getting hotter and hotter... and hotter. Eventually, she woke up in severe pain and with second-degree burns to her inner thigh and one side of her vagina.

In his 1922 book *Rovering To Success*, Lord Baden-Powell – founder of the Boy Scout movement – warned young boys on the dangers of masturbation, claiming, 'It cheats semen [of] getting its full chance of making up the strong manly man you would otherwise be.' It's not certain whether he practised what he preached, as Baden-Powell is reported to have liked looking at photos of nude schoolboys with a schoolmaster friend, who was a keen amateur photographer of his pupils.

In November 2012 police were called to a Florida Starbucks after receiving reports of a woman openly masturbating in the coffee shop. A police spokesman commented, 'No one could ever say for sure what she was doing, and I'm pretty sure the video didn't show anything definitive but her hands went into her pants when she was wigging out.' The accused, twenty-nine-year-old, Jennifer Piranian, told officers she wasn't well due to 'an infection or spider bite.'

A woman who was admitted to a Leningrad hospital with glass splinters in her vagina finally confessed to doctors that she had been masturbating with a cylinder-shaped light bulb that broke when she was using it. The girl usually used a warm bulb in a lamp to increase her pleasure. Fortunately for her, in this case, she hadn't switched it on.

A phone-sex operator in Florida won a large settlement after filing for worker's compensation, claiming she had suffered repetitive-strain injuries in both hands. This was the result of giving herself as many as seven orgasms a day while talking to clients.

In the 1880s castration was sometimes prescribed as a cure for serious masturbators. A contemporary account about one American patient claimed that, after the operation, he was 'cheerful and happy' and had, at last, 'the prospect of good health and a life of usefulness.'

Poet Edward Lear blamed his epileptic fits on his over-zealous fondness for masturbation.

In many prisons, gardening duty is popular among inmates. Not because it gives them a chance to work outdoors but because many of them use the opportunity to collect worms, which they put into a jam jar. Back in their cells, each prisoner slightly warms the jar on a radiator and inserts his penis into the jar, using it as a masturbatory device.

In the 1890s some authorities believed that women could be aroused by riding bicycles. The *Georgia Journal of Medicine and Surgery* claimed that 'the pedalling machine' could cause 'undesirable gynaecological effects, especially when the body is thrown forward, causing the clothing to press against the clitoris, thereby eliciting and arousing feelings hitherto unknown and unrealised by the young maiden.'

For similar reasons, in France, the *Académie de Medicine* protested against the sewing machine.

The *Medical Aspects of Human Sexuality Journal* of July 1991 contains a story of an unmarried factory worker and self-confessed 'bit of a loner' who had taken to masturbating against the canvas-belt drive of a piece of machinery where he worked. One day a momentary lapse of concentration caused his scrotum to be caught between the drive belt and the pulley wheel. The man was knocked unconscious as he was drawn into the machinery and, when he awoke, discovered his left testicle missing. To close the wound, he used the most convenient thing to hand – an industrial staple gun.

IS IT IN YET?

The author of the article, Dr Gavin Matthews, who examined the man, stated that the testicle was never found and said, 'I can only assume he abandoned this method of self-gratification.'

As a deterrent against masturbation, Chinese authorities used to recommend 'Hard study of the works of Marx, Lenin and Chairman Mao.'

In 1897 Dr John Harvey Kellogg invented the cornflakes that share his name as an 'anti-masturbation food'. Kellogg was a fervent crusader against the perils of masturbation and believed a meat-free breakfast would reduce the prevalence of this heinous act. If this failed to have the desired effect, he recommended sewing up boys' foreskins with silver wire.

Spectators at Toronto's baseball stadium found it difficult to keep their eye on the ball during a Blue Jays–Seattle Mariners game in the early 1990s. They were distracted by one of the guests staying at the Skydome Hotel, which is visible from inside the stadium. This particular guest apparently thought the windows were made of one-way glass and several thousand fans saw him standing at the window of his room, masturbating while he watched the game.

GOING SOLO

Commenting on the great view the hotel affords over the stadium, the manager commented, 'There isn't a more exciting way to watch a baseball game but, for some people, it's more exciting than for others.'

British birth-control pioneer Marie Stopes didn't know what masturbation was until she was twenty-nine.

To discourage masturbation among boys and young men in the Victorian era, there were a whole host of ingenious inventions available that were a cross between chastity belts and torture devices. Many were featured in the contemporary best-selling catalogue *Spermatorrhea*. This included genital cages and penis rings lined with spikes and even an intricate device that rang a bell located in the parents' room when their son had an erection.

An 1897 book, *What A Young Boy Should Know*, stated that masturbation 'causes idiocy and even death' and cited examples of boys being put in straitjackets or having their hands tied to rings in the wall in order to discourage this heinous act.

In ancient times, men would masturbate on the altars in pagan churches. Depositing semen was seen as the ultimate gift to the gods.

IS IT IN YET?

Also in the distant past, Jewish rabbis forbade men from holding their penises during urination, in case it encouraged them to masturbate.

A thirty-three-year-old Swansea woman went shopping to her local Asda supermarket wearing her new Ann Summers 'Passion Pants', which contained a 2.5-inch 'vibrating bullet' inside them. Such was the intensity of the pleasure that the happy shopper fainted and banged her head on a display, knocking herself out in the process. The reason for her accident became apparent when paramedics detected the still-buzzing panties on arrival and disabled them, returning them discreetly to their grateful owner after she'd recovered.

In 1992 newspapers reported that an unnamed thirty-two-year-old woman became convinced that Donald Duck was in love with her, via signals beamed to her from her neighbour's satellite dish.

The neighbour found her standing near the dish, masturbating, convinced that Donald was simultaneously making love to her.

AWKWARD MOMENTS

Sex itself shouldn't be embarrassing but it can be when any form of discretion is disregarded. Like the time a man presented himself at his local ER with a mobile phone firmly jammed up his bottom, or when a cameraman left a scene of himself 'entertaining' a bull terrier on a bride's wedding video...

In May 1994, hearing what were described as 'blood curdling' screams coming from a house in Reading, Berkshire, neighbours immediately called the police. Officers arrived within minutes and broke into the house but there was no murder in progress – just a deaf couple having sex. The passionate couple had removed their hearing aids and had no idea how loud they were shouting.

IS IT IN YET?

When Antonio Mendoza arrived at a Los Angeles ER with a mobile phone firmly wedged up his rectum, he said he had a bona fide reason for how it had happened. Apparently, Mendoza's dog had taken his phone into the shower and he was so surprised that he slipped over, the dog had dropped the phone and he'd landed right on top of it. The medics were not convinced of his story but managed to retrieve the phone, which rang three times during the delicate extraction operation.

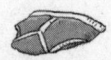

Twenty-year-old Daisy Gladden was hospitalised for hypothermia after spending four days trapped in a freezing car underneath a man she'd just had sex with. The man had died but Daisy told her rescuers, 'I just thought he was a heavy sleeper.'

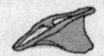

A couple from San Jose called the emergency services after a freak accident made them unable to separate during sex. One of the man's testicles had slid inside his girlfriend and, taken by surprise, the girl got scared, which involuntarily closed her vagina. The result was that the man's orphaned testicle and his penis were locked inside her. An application of muscle relaxant came to the rescue and, apart from a bruised testicle, all was, once again, back to normal.

AWKWARD MOMENTS

A man who presented himself to A&E with his swollen penis stuck in the end of a ring spanner admitted that he had been masturbating with it. Staff tried to drain blood but the penis was held fast. As a last resort, the fire brigade were called and they used an industrial hacksaw to remove the offending tool (the spanner, that is). According to the duty nurse, sparks were flying everywhere and they had to coat the victim's penis in cream to stop it getting burned. She commented that, during the lengthy procedure, all the man could say was, 'I'm sorry. I'm so, so sorry!'

French president Félix Francois Faure died suddenly in the Élysée Palace in 1899 at the hand — or rather, the mouth — of his younger lover. Reports at the time stated that he'd suffered a fatal seizure while engaging in fellatio with Mme Margueritte Steinheil. So shocked was she at his demise that she developed lockjaw and his penis had to be carefully prized out of her mouth. Among her circle of friends and acquaintances, Steinheil was later known by the ignoble nickname 'pompe funèbre', which can be translated literally as 'funeral blow-job'.

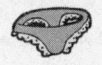

In March 2003, when *The Sun* revealed that former Welsh Secretary Ron Davies had taken part in a sex act in broad daylight on Tog Hill near Bath, the politician claimed that all he was doing there was looking for badgers.

IS IT IN YET?

Film of a 1994 Sussex wedding reception had a few surprises for the guests who'd sat down to watch the happy event. At the end of the video, they saw the owner of the video camera – fifty-nine-year-old Derek Jeffrey – wearing nothing but his socks and taking part in unusual and unnatural acts with a Staffordshire bull terrier called Ronnie. He'd forgotten to erase the tape. He was found guilty of bestiality with a dog but was remanded on bail for psychiatric reports.

In a case of mistaken identity, a hairdresser in Christchurch, New Zealand who was working late became concerned when her client began making brisk pumping motions under the hairdresser's cape he was wearing. Alone in the salon and terrified she was in the presence of a pervert, she hit him hard over the head, rendering him unconscious, then called the police.

It was later found that all the innocent man had been doing was cleaning his glasses.

From time to time, Donald Thompson, fifty-nine – a former Creek County, Oklahoma district judge – seemed distracted during various hearings. The cause was soon apparent. Under his judicial robes, he was masturbating using a penis pump. One witness said she saw him expose himself fifteen to twenty times and lost count of the times she'd heard a 'shhh-shhh' noise from under his robes, while nine former jurors testified they heard pumping noises coming from the judge. At his trial, it was also claimed that, as well as using the pump, the judge also oiled and shaved his genitals during trials.

Thompson admitted having the penis pump but insisted it was a joke gift from a pal for his fiftieth birthday. He was convicted on four counts of indecent exposure, arising from four jury trials in 2002 and 2003, and a year behind bars plus a fine for each offence was recommended.

Lisa Foster – a court reporter – commented that the judge had even masturbated while hearing evidence from the grandfather of a murdered toddler, saying, 'The grandfather was getting real teary-eyed and the judge was up there pumping.'

Police Sergeant Michael Reed, who testified as a witness, commented, 'This repeated use of a penis pump while performing his judicial duties violated the requirement that judges personally observe a high standard of conduct.'

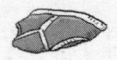

Ivan and Valentina Sokolov – a Russian couple in their fifties – had just received a copy of the *Kama Sutra* and decided to use it to add a little spice into their sex life. Unfortunately, the position they chose – the Indrani or 'deck chair' position – was one of the more complicated ones and involved 'the woman drawing up her knees so her feet are jammed under her partner's armpits'. All was going well until Valentina climaxed and triggered a muscle spasm that trapped Ivan's penis inside her.

After trying, unsuccessfully, to separate themselves for two hours, they eventually decided to call an ambulance. The couple were later separated in hospital.

A Welshman sued an amateur hypnotist who put him a trance in June 1993 and got him to make love to a chair, much to the amusement of all the audience. The problem was that the hypnotist was alleged to have accidentally failed to wake the man properly from the trance and, as a result, the victim found himself compelled to simulate sex with a whole host of objects and appliances at home, including his mattress, washing machine, tumble drier, every chair in his house and even his bath. The case came to court but later collapsed due to inconsistencies in the evidence.

A woman in south-west England called the police after receiving a phone call from her daughter in the early hours of the morning. It sounded like she was in a state of real distress; the woman could hear what sounded like the sounds of a struggle, a man's muffled voice and her daughter yelling, 'Oh my God!' several times before the line when dead. Fearing the worst, the woman called the local police, who went round to investigate, only to discover that the daughter had been engrossed in some really passionate sex with her boyfriend, whose toe had been accidentally hitting the autodial button on the bedside phone.

AWKWARD MOMENTS

A middle-aged woman in England, who lived alone, was woken by a strange noise in her house and, fearing an intruder, immediately called the police. Officers arrived and searched the house and, according to reports, once they found the source of the sound, the woman's face went from 'white with fear to red with embarrassment'. A spokesman for the police said the officers on call had difficulty keeping a straight face when they realised it was a vibrator on her bedside table that had somehow been accidentally switched on.

Forty-two-year-old Daniel Blackner – AKA 'Captain Dan the Demon Dwarf' – was rushed to hospital after accidentally gluing his penis to a Henry vacuum cleaner. The incident happened as he prepared for a show at the Edinburgh Fringe Festival in August 2007. As part of his act, Captain Dan pulls the vacuum cleaner across the stage attached to his penis but, on this occasion, the attachment connecting the dwarf to the appliance came loose. Deciding to fix it himself, he failed to wait for the extra-strong glue to dry. This meant that, when he reinserted his penis, he was immediately stuck fast.

Dan was rushed to Edinburgh Royal Infirmary, where, he said, nurses struggled for an hour to free him. He commented, 'It was the most embarrassing moment of my life when I got wheeled into a packed A&E with a vacuum attached to me. I just wished the ground could swallow me up. Luckily, they saw me quickly, so the embarrassment was short-lived.'

IS IT IN YET?

Dr Harvey White – one of New Zealand's leading cardiologists – was sacked from his $200,000-a-year position by Auckland City Hospital in May 2005 after emailing photos of his penis to staff. The pictures were discovered by administration staff, who reported the doctor to hospital authorities. The Employment Court heard how Dr White had taken pictures on his cell phone in the toilet at home before downloading them onto his work computer. However, he told the hearing that he'd just been 'trying to imitate a television commercial.'

Dr White was eventually reinstated to his post six months later, after successfully appealing against his sacking. During the hearing, Supreme Court Judge Graham Colgan said White's actions were 'bizarre and inappropriate.'

Drug addict Nicki Jex held up a Ladbrokes betting shop in Leicester in December 2006 by pointing a gun concealed in a carrier bag at the terrified cashier. She handed over everything that was in her till – a total of £613 – and Jex fled. The only customer in the shop at the time bravely followed him out but Jex waved the gun, yelling at him to back off. Unknown to the raider, Jex was followed to a local pub, where he was arrested by police. To everyone's surprise (apart from the thief), the 'gun' in the bag turned out to be his girlfriend's 'Rampant Rabbit' vibrator. Jex was jailed for five years for robbery.

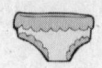

AWKWARD MOMENTS

Belt buckles and penises don't mix, as a Bristol man found to his horror in December 1987. During sex games, his wife had slid the heavy brass buckle over his penis, where it became stuck. The more she tried to pull it off, the more his penis became swollen, making removal impossible. In the end, the man drove to the nearest fire station with the belt still attached to his manhood. Unable to remove it, the firemen drove the man to Bristol Royal infirmary, where doctors were more successful.

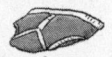

In 2001 an unnamed American man turned up at his local ER and, after a brief examination, was sent through to see a doctor with the acronym FBIP on his notes. This is ER shorthand for Foreign Body In Penis but, in this case, the subsequent examination showed not one but two foreign objects. The first was a length of aquarium tubing and the second was a long length of thin nylon cord – the type used in lawn trimmers. The embarrassed patient told the doctor that he wanted to see what would happen if he inserted a three-foot length of plastic tubing into his penis. He'd managed to insert most of it when it became firmly stuck. In a futile – and idiotic – attempt to try and remove it, he threaded the nylon cord through the middle, only to find that this, too, became lodged.

The man hoped that the objects would come lose on their own... but they didn't. Subsequent X-rays revealed that both objects had become kinked and lodged in his bladder and careful surgery was required to remove them. The man blamed marijuana for his experimentation.

IS IT IN YET?

When US Immigration officials searched Ahmed Mustafa's luggage, they were horrified to discover a 'grenade-like' object. Mustafa was in a quandary: should he risk admitting to carrying a penis pump? He decided the shame would be too great so, instead, he said it was a bomb. The authorities were far from amused and he was charged with the felony of 'disorderly conduct'.

An off-duty St Louis policeman heard sustained screams from his neighbours' home. Fearing the worst, he broke in, gun drawn, to provide assistance. Naked and tied to her bed was the neighbour. Lying unconscious on the floor was her husband, dressed as Batman. The couple had been acting out a role-paying fantasy whereby the husband was supposed to jump off the top of a wardrobe to 'save' his wife. Except he missed and knocked himself out after hitting the floor.

In October 2014 an anonymous Italian couple took advantage of a warm day and deserted beach by stripping off and having sex in the sea in the Marche region to the northeast of the country. A very enjoyable experience soon came to an awkward end when the couple realised they couldn't separate. The Italian newspaper *Il Mattino* reported that the man 'was unable to extricate himself from the woman due to suction.' Carefully manoeuvring themselves on to the beach 'still as one', the couple were only able to separate after being taken to hospital, where a doctor gave the woman an injection to dilate her womb.

Police called to a Florida Hotel by the desk clerk, who reported that one of the guests was 'stuck in the pool', did not expect to find thirty-year-old Stephen Drummond with his swimming trunks pulled down and his penis caught in one of the pool's suction inlets. Drummond's penis had become so swollen in his attempts to pull himself free that shutting off the pump had no effect. Eventually, he was released after a copious amount of lubricant was poured over the suction fitting.

Feeling sorry for Drummond, the police declined to prosecute him. Officer Mel Johnson commented that 'There's no law covering unlawful sexual intercourse with a rubber chlorinator nozzle.' The press found out about the incident but, in a statement, Drummond tried to play down what had happened, saying, 'It's the sort of thing that could happen to anyone.'

Workers at a Berlin post office began panicking when a package began vibrating and making 'strange noises'. The police were called and, tracing the sender, immediately rushed round to arrest who they thought was a bomb-maker. The man they questioned was actually innocent of any terrorist charges. He was just a normal Joe but one who was returning

IS IT IN YET?

a life-sized sex doll to the manufacturers. This model had a vibrating vagina that was faulty; it would spontaneously turn itself on at the most inopportune times... like in the post office.

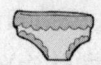

JUST PLAIN STUPID

There's the woman who cut off her husband's penis in order to restore the passion in their marriage, the man who attempted sex with a hedgehog and the guy who shot himself in the groin so his ex-girlfriend would feel sorry for him. Whoever said, 'Never underestimate the power of human stupidity,' certainly knew what they were talking about.

Errol Glover of Hampden County Massachusetts thought of the perfect way to trick his identical twin brother's girlfriend into having sex with him. One night, when his brother was out, he crept into bed with the girlfriend, knowing it would be impossible for her to tell them apart physically. Errol would have got away with it had he not forgotten her name.

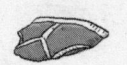

IS IT IN YET?

A peeping Tom in Colar, France drilled a small hole in his wall so he could observe his next-door neighbours in bed. Unfortunately, he got so excited watching them make love that he had to light up a cigarette... the smoke drifted into their bedroom through the peephole and alerted his angry neighbours.

A man who visited his local A&E department surprised the medics on duty. Not because he had a vacuum cleaner attachment fixed to his penis but because, rather than just detach the hose beforehand, he came in dragging the whole vacuum cleaner with him – drawing even more attention to himself.

Sandy Kroll of Corio, Australia had been stalking a local woman and bombarding her with sexually explicit phone calls and videos of him masturbating almost non-stop over a seven-day period. In all cases, his own phone number was withheld. The worried woman reported him to the police and, as she was filing a complaint at the police station, he rang once again. This time, the sophisticated police equipment easily traced the call and the anonymous masturbator was arrested.

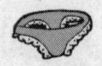

JUST PLAIN STUPID

In 2001 Stephen Millhouse of Cedar Rapids, Iowa broke into a woman's apartment and, after she woke up, he asked her for sex. In a state of shock, but staying clam, she declined his offer. Millhouse then asked the woman for a proper date and, to get him out of her house, she agreed. They met and he was arrested by police lying in wait. During the trial, Millhouse's lawyers claimed their client was too stupid to be dangerous. The jury disagreed and he was convicted of burglary in the second degree.

Serbian Zoran Nikolovic, thirty-five, of Belgrade required emergency surgery after attempting to have sex with a large hedgehog. The hedgehog was apparently unharmed after its ordeal; a hospital spokesman commented, 'The patient came off much worse from the encounter.'

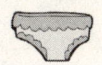

Putting your penis between two slices of bread in the presence of a large dog isn't the brightest thing to do, as a Staffordshire policeman found to his cost in January 1995. Thinking he could entice his wife into some morning sex, he presented his 'penis sandwich' to her in the kitchen. Before she could react, the family's Labrador leaped up at what he perceived was a breakfast treat. The result was that the officer was off work for several days and required cosmetic surgery to repair the damage. When asked for a statement on the foolhardy actions of their colleague, a spokesman for the police said,

IS IT IN YET?

'We couldn't possibly comment on what a police officer does in his spare time.'

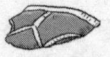

A Sicilian man in the town of Piazza Amerina was admitted to hospital with a shotgun wound to his groin. At first he claimed this was the result of a hunting accident but later changed his story when doctors became suspicious. He admitted that he wanted to get back with his ex-girlfriend and thought the best way to do this was to get her to feel sorry for him. The way he did this was to get one of his friends to shoot him in the groin. All was in vain, however. Local reports stated that the ex-girlfriend said she never wanted to see him again.

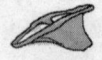

Fuelled by beer and a high degree of lust, a man removed a stripper's panties with his mouth but then accidentally swallowed them. He waited for the panties to pass through but they didn't emerge. Instead, he just felt unwell and bloated. Rather than seek medical advice at this stage, the man then decided to try some DIY surgery and, making a hook from an old wire coat hanger, tried to fish them out by poking it deep down inside his throat. Instead of snagging the panties, all he managed to do was rip large gashes along the length of his oesophagus and he subsequently died from the effects of a massive infection.

JUST PLAIN STUPID

Martin – a thirty-four-year-old Englishman – frequently asked his wife to smother him with her nightie while they had sex. Alone one day, he decided to take the whole 'suffocation thing' up a notch and put a plastic bag over his head, before using a vacuum cleaner to remove the air. Unfortunately, he removed too much... His wife found him dead, next to the still-running Hoover.

During his stag night at a strip club in Fort Wayne, Indiana, in May 2003, Justin Scheidt consented to take the stage and lay on his back with his legs around the dance pole, while several strippers slid down on to his crotch. Afterwards, he sued the club, as he suffered 'serious and permanent injuries' to his groin. He went ahead with his wedding but claimed he was unable to consummate the marriage.

An American woman sued her local pharmacy for $1 million after she bought a contraceptive jelly and, despite using it daily, still managed to get pregnant. She claimed she wasn't given the appropriate advice over its application... it turned out that she was spreading it on her toast.

In July 2000 twenty-somethings Elizabeth Whitaker and Aaron Caudhill decided to get amorous in an amusement-

IS IT IN YET?

park photo booth in Mason, Ohio, not realising that the photos taken were also displayed on a screen outside the booth – in this case, of Elizabeth performing oral sex. When Aaron realised the images were in full public view, he rushed out to try and cover the screen with his hands. The couple were arrested on charges of public indecency. A spokesman commented, 'We're a family park and try to operate and maintain a family experience.'

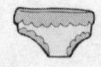

A San Diego man known only as Shaun attempted to get into his married lover's home by climbing down the chimney, only to get stuck in the narrow shaft twelve feet from the top. His cries alerted neighbours, who called the police. Shaun was wedged so tight that he couldn't be pulled free by ropes; the only way of freeing him was to knock a hole in the chimney from inside the house. This noisy demolition – and the horde of reporters who surrounded him on his liberation – destroyed any hope of trying to keep his visit discreet.

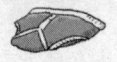

Dutchman Peter Koenings was deported back to his home country for harassing women travelling by bus in Nottingham. He would climb under seats and tickle them with his long tongue, which he'd stick through the small gap between cushions. It didn't take police too long to arrest him – he used the same bus each time.

JUST PLAIN STUPID

Two women in the heat of passion were distraught when the strap of their strap-on dildo broke after some very energetic sex. Not wanting to lose the moment, they looked around the house for a replacement and the nearest thing they could find was the plunger kept under the kitchen sink. They pondered on how to attach it, and then one of them then had the not-very-bright idea of using superglue. The nurse who had to subsequently remove it had this to say about a plunger stuck to the vagina: 'It's very hard to hide whether you are sitting, lying or standing in the waiting room of A&E.'

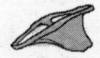

A man from Wauwatosa, Wisconsin received a citation for disorderly conduct after being found guilty in 1995 of entering the women's toilets in the town's Mayfair Mall. In his defence, he claimed he just did it because he thought it would be a good way to meet women.

Michael Guilbault, nineteen, and an accomplice robbed a convenience store in Raleigh, North Carolina but found themselves locked out of their getaway car while two other gang members, Heather Beckwith and Curtis Johnson, had sex on the back seat. Guilbault's impatient pounding on the car and yelling attracted onlookers and the gang was arrested.

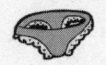

IS IT IN YET?

In 1994 a Chinese housewife consulted a soothsayer to find out how she could restore the passion in her marriage. Acting on his advice, she then cut off her husband's penis while he slept, only to discover that the soothsayer had lied – he didn't grow a new one.

An Ohio man found that an element of danger increased his sexual satisfaction, so he'd tie himself to railway tracks and masturbate, timing his climax to just before the train arrived. The last time he did this was the day it took him longer than usual to get aroused and he couldn't untie himself in time.

Believe it or not, there is definitely such a thing as too much sex, as twenty-eight-year-old Russian Sergey Tuganov discovered. He bet two women the equivalent of about £3,000 that he could have sex with them both for twelve hours non-stop. To assist in this marathon, he took Viagra… but not just one or two tablets. Tuganov gulped down a whole bottle and died of a sudden heart attack.

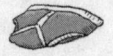

Romanian Nicolae Popoci, a father of five, didn't want any more children, so he devised a sure-fire way of ensuring his condom wouldn't fall off during lovemaking: superglue. It wasn't until after having sex that he realised the condom was

JUST PLAIN STUPID

stuck fast. He and his wife tried various methods to remove it with no luck, so they went to the local medical clinic for help. He told nurses that a benefit of having the condom stuck to his penis was that could use it again later.

Agata Wisniewski and her lover James Rogers were engrossed in a kinky 'cops and robbers' sex game when Wisniewski accidentally fired a shot that hit Rogers in the head, killing him instantly. Police believed the woman's story about the sex game gone wrong and charged her with negligent homicide – a lesser crime than murder.

A Thai construction worker in Bahrain was so overwrought on hearing the news that his wife had left him that he decided to make a real statement about his feelings. He cut off his own penis.

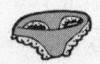

In September 1999 Ron Guptey of New South Wales was forced to go to his local A&E department, complaining of a raging fever and a severe pain in his rectum. Unsure if the two conditions were connected, doctors admitted him to hospital for observation, where he fell into a coma and died the next day. An autopsy revealed that a black widow spider had laid eggs in Ron's rectum. Once the baby spiders were

IS IT IN YET?

hatched, they had bitten him and had poisoned him from the inside. What puzzled medics the most was how they'd got there? The answer came from the post-mortem, which revealed traces of tree bark and KY jelly in Ron's rectum. He'd apparently been satisfying himself with a tree stump in his garden but had failed to notice the black-widow nest.

Peeping Toms normally press their faces against the glass of a ground or first-floor window; not one twelve storeys up. That's what Japanese serial voyeur Tadao Tanaka did in 1999, climbing on to a woman's balcony for a night of peeping, only to slip and plunge to his death.

One S&M aficionado wanted to avoid injury during a sex role-play game, so he made sure the knife he gave his girlfriend wasn't too sharp. Unfortunately, her role was that of a Nazi hangman, while he played the victim. Tragedy occurred when she hanged him and then tried to cut him down; the knife was too blunt to cut the noose and he was strangled.

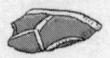

In December 1988 two new workers at an aluminium plant in Slatina, Romania decided that the high-pressure hoses used to power industrial air tools had another obvious use:

JUST PLAIN STUPID

to blow air across their testicles. If their thrills had stopped there, all would have been OK. Instead, one of the men decided to insert the hose into his rectum and release six bars of pressure.

The autopsy revealed that the worker had completely ruptured several metres of his colon and intestines – as well as breaking factory regulations.

In June 1987 a thirty-four-year-old New York man decided to inject cocaine directly into his urethra in order to enhance his sexual performance. The consequences were both good and bad. The immediate benefit was a three-day erection. The downside was that, after the third day, the erection suddenly subsided but, over the next twelve hours, blood leaked into the tissues of his feet, hands, genitals, back and chest. The coagulation caused tissues to die over large areas of the patient's body and he was transferred to the burns unit of New York-Presbyterian Hospital/Weill Cornell Medical Center. There, doctors were forced to amputate the man's legs above the knee and nine of his fingers to stop the spread of gangrene. It was reported that the patient's penis fell off by itself.

After being missing for thirty-six hours, a boy-scout leader from Florida was eventually found by a search party, naked (apart from his shoes) and hanging upside down from a tree by a rope tied around one of his ankles. Police also found a video camera trained on him. Investigators found that the man had intended to film an 'autoerotic situation' but that something had gone very wrong and he was left suspended by one foot, twelve feet from the ground. A lack of circulation meant that this foot had to be amputated. An officer of the Sheriff's Department astutely commented, 'Some things are better confined to your own home.'

When an unnamed Pakistani patient turned up at the hospital to explain what a Coca-Cola bottle was doing up his rectum, he must have thought the doctor on duty was particularly dim. The reason he gave was that 'Thieves inserted it up my bottom and then ran away.'

A man from Toronto decided to take his kitchen sink apart and insert his penis into the trash-disposal unit. Despite suffering life-changing injuries from the blades, the man managed to call the emergency services. When asked by horrified doctors why he had carried out this act, he calmly said, 'I wanted to see what it felt like.'

It takes a true idiot to mistake a shop mannequin for a sex doll but that's exactly what happened when an unnamed

JUST PLAIN STUPID

man complained to Displaysense – the shop-dummy manufacturers – after getting his penis painfully stuck in a 24 mm hole designed for a display stand. A spokesman for the company commented, 'We will now warn people that our mannequins are for display use only and not for recreational use.'

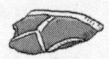

Looking for a new sexual thrill, in May 2007 thirty-one-year-old Gary Ashbrook from Newhaven, East Sussex inflated a condom with laughing gas and put it over his head. He suffocated.

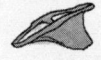

BEASTLY BEHAVIOUR

For some people, a dog is more than their best friend – it's their lover. However, some people believe there's no reason to stop at dogs when there's a whole menagerie of animals just waiting to be seduced, including dolphins, eels, elephants, monkeys and even an octopus. Two legs are good – but, according to these stories, no legs, four legs or eight arms are better.

Timothy Bodkins was fined $750 for having sex with a turkey at the poultry plant where he worked in Adams County, Pennsylvania. He admitted assaulting the 20-lb bird but told police that he only did it when two co-workers made it worth his while; he sodomised the turkey for $12 and three packets of chewing gum.

IS IT IN YET?

Police suspected forty-nine-year-old Bradley Brainard, from Atascadero, California, of selling drugs to prison inmates at the California Men's Colony, where he had been working as a plumber on a construction project. However, they came across something really unexpected when they searched his house in April 2009: a video showing him 'on a bed, naked, wearing a woman's brassiere, alongside a chocolate Labrador', performing various sexual acts. Brainard later commented, 'It's something I got into that I never should have gotten into.'

In a short film called *Dolphin Lover*, Malcolm Brenner, sixty-three, admits to having a sexual relationship with a dolphin called Dolly in 1971 but only because she seduced him. At the time of the relationship, which lasted a year, Mr Brenner was a photographer who had access to a theme park in Sarasota, Florida. He was given free access to the dolphins and says the affair began when he started going swimming with her, saying, 'She announced her intentions to me by positioning herself so I was rubbing against her.' Having sex with Dolly didn't break any laws, since bestiality was only banned in Florida in 1971. The nine-month relationship ended when the theme park closed and Dolly was re-homed. In the film, Mr Brenner also admitted to having previous sexual experiences with a dog.

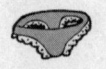

BEASTLY BEHAVIOUR

Sixty-one-year-old Kim Lee Chong was sentenced to fifteen years in prison by a court in Phuket, Thailand after being convicted for attempting to have sex with an elephant. He'd been caught standing on a box behind the beast, naked from the waist down. At his hearing, Chong claimed the elephant was the reincarnation of his dead wife, explaining, 'I recognised her immediately by the naughty glint in her eyes.'

I'm not sure if this story should go in this section or the section titled 'That's Just Wrong!' (or even in a special new one called 'Just Stop It, Now!'). In 2008 a Tasmanian man was caught downloading images of a very niche type of sexual act – those involving humans having sex with octopuses. His lawyer explained that his client's self-esteem was 'so low'.

Police announced that they were seeking a man who'd been observed touching the genitals of a twelve-foot long bottle-nosed dolphin off the pier in the fishing town of Amble, Northumberland. Marine zoologist Peter Bloom noticed injuries on the dolphin's penis that he concluded were the result of someone encouraging the animal to 'use it unnaturally.'

Commenting on a different case involving Fungie – a wild dolphin at Dingle Bay Harbour, Kerry, Ireland – the zoologist said, 'I saw a stark-naked woman run into the sea

IS IT IN YET?

shouting, "Come on, Fungie I love you." Dolphins bring out the best and worst in people.'

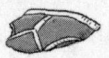

It was a case of 'bear-faced cheek' when a Devon man applied for a job at a Barnstaple animal sanctuary, only to be refused the post when staff interviewing him recognised his photo from the local newspaper. He'd recently been arrested for molesting animals while working at a local zoo.

Two British workers in Algeria thought they were being hilarious when they simulated sex with a herd of sheep in the eastern town of Hassi Messaoud. Locals never do find this sort of thing amusing but, on this occasion, they were absolutely incensed. The sheep in question were lined up to be slaughtered for the sacred Muslim festival of Eid. The two workers were sacked.

Someone with absolutely no shame was Paulo 'Chico' Lopez of Valencia, Spain, who had sex with a bull in the middle of the city's main bullring in front of 20,000 cheering spectators. It was later reported that he managed to achieve success 'after several unsuccessful attempts and some nasty kicks.'

BEASTLY BEHAVIOUR

A seventy-two-year-old man sexually abused a pig on a London urban farm. Police thought he'd been planning his attack for a while, as he specifically chose the farm's most docile pig. The farm owner commented, 'If he'd picked on one of the others, he would have been in serious trouble. They would have done him some damage.'

A British lorry driver from Leicester pleaded guilty in February 2008 of having sex with a variety of dogs between 1974 and 2004. Police were alerted by his son, who found a video of his father with a black Labrador and a mongrel. Admitting the indecent acts, the lorry driver claimed that he'd been trying to erase them from his memory, as he knew that what he had done 'wasn't quite right.'

In October 2008 Carol Hickey – a forty-three-year-old mother of four from Limerick, Ireland – had sex with a dog (an Alsatian) for the first time but died soon afterwards from a severe allergic reaction to the dog's semen.

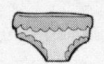

In August 1996 a man from Eagleville, Tennessee was arrested for having sex with a miniature horse. On discovering there was no law that applied to having sex with animals, the court could only charge the man with indecent exposure.

IS IT IN YET?

An unnamed women inserted a live eel into her vagina for stimulation. Whether or not it had the desired effect was unreported, although, as a result, she did receive a vaginal infection.

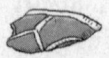

Missouri resident Mark Mathews loved his horse Pixie so much that he not only had sex with her, he married her too and even made her lingerie. Mark featured on the 1999 UK documentary *Hidden Love: Animal Passions* and also in an episode of *The Jerry Springer Show* the year before, titled 'I Married A Horse'. The show was, ultimately, not aired by many stations on the planned date, due to concerns about its 'suitability'.

Frederick the Great, who it was said never slept with his wife, was rumoured to have been romantically linked with his pack of whippet bitches.

There are numerous reports of amorous (and brave) Egyptian men having sex with female crocodiles, taking advantage of the fact that, once on her back, the creature finds it quite difficult to right herself.

BEASTLY BEHAVIOUR

A few years ago a New Zealand judge sentenced a man to seven years in prison for having sex with a sheep. He then suspended the sentence, explaining to the jury that, 'Society no longer frowns on sex with a sheep.'

In Peru, it's illegal for an unmarried man to share his house with a female llama.

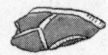

There are many reports of lonely women in rural communities sprinkling gains of barley over their vaginas and encouraging geese or chickens to peck them off.

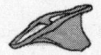

Until April 2015 Denmark had no specific bestiality laws, which meant that, as long as animals were not harmed, it was legal for humans to have sex with them. This had previously given rise to a burgeoning animal-sex tourism industry and a number of secret animal bordellos, where people paid to have sex with horses, cows, sheep and llamas.

It's customary for women of the Trukese tribe in Micronesia to place coconut in their vaginas and then to have a dog lick it out.

IS IT IN YET?

In February 2006 a Sudanese man, Charles Tombe, was caught having sex with a neighbour's goat and ordered by the council of elders to pay the neighbour a dowry to the equivalent of $75 and marry the animal.

In 1981 a Moroccan man, Abdel Brim Talal, was attacked by angry locals after sexually assaulting a pelican, which was the mascot of the Greek island of Tinos. The bird was found in a public toilet and Talal found it difficult to claim he was unconnected with the crime – he was found nearby covered with blood and feathers.

Until 2011 there were no anti-bestiality laws in Florida. In 2005 a man charged with having sex with his dog could only be charged with disorderly conduct.

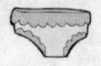

A male employee at San Antonio Zoo told staff at Sea World of Texas that he wanted to work there 'so he could have sex with a dolphin.' The man admitted to having sex with cats, dogs, horses, sheep, goats, cows, a duck, a pig, a gazelle and a baboon in 1985.

He did not get the job.

BEASTLY BEHAVIOUR

If male or female members of the Kurtachi tribe of the Solomon Islands can't find a mate, they consider it perfectly acceptable to have sex with a dog instead.

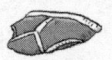

In West Virginia it's legal for a man to have sex with an animal as long as it does not exceed 40 lbs.

In March 1995 an unnamed Zimbabwe man was charged with having sex with a cow. At his court appearance, he declared that he was in love with the cow, recited marriage vows from the dock and pledged that he'd be faithful to the animal while serving his sentence. He got nine months.

A night watchman doing his rounds in Botswana heard what he thought was the sound of screeching brakes, only to discover that it was the noise of a braying donkey. The reason was soon apparent – a man behind it, having sex with the animal. When challenged, the man just said in his defence that the donkey didn't mind and that, anyway, it was his own donkey.

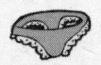

IS IT IN YET?

Thomas Aloysius McCarney, from south Galway, checked into a hotel with a donkey, registering his companion as 'Mr Shrek'. Receptionist Irina Legova said that Mr McCarney had told her that the donkey was a breed of 'super rabbit', which he was bringing to a pet fair in the city – and she believed him. However, she had reason to question her naivety when the donkey was found running berserk though the hotel in the middle of the night and its absent owner discovered wearing a latex suit, handcuffed to his bed, the donkey having swallowed the key. Mr McCarney was arrested and charged with animal cruelty and lewd and obscene behaviour. A further charge of damaging the mini-bar was dropped after McCarney explained it was the donkey, rather than him, that was responsible.

According to news reports, the original charges were dropped and he was eventually fined €2,000 (approx. £1,350) for bringing the donkey to the room under the Unlawful Accommodation of Donkeys Act 1837.

Victorian poet Algernon Charles Swinburne (1837–1909) admitted having sexual relations with a monkey that was dressed as a woman.

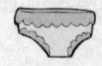

Sculptor and graphic designer Eric Gill, who designed the classically elegant typeface 'Gill Sans' in 1926, recorded in his own diaries various sex acts performed on his own dog.

BEASTLY BEHAVIOUR

This aspect of his life was deliberately omitted from his 1966 biography but added in a 1989 version, at which point it became public knowledge.

Kenneth Pinyan of Enumclaw, Washington State took horsing around a bit further than he should have. In July 2005 he was filmed by a friend engaging in receptive anal sex with an Arab stallion on a farm in King County. A short while later, Pinyan was anonymously dropped off at Enumclaw Community Hospital by someone who told doctors he needed 'medical attention'. He died a short while later from a perforated colon in the emergency room.

The video soon found its way on to the Internet and was one of the most read stories in the area's newspaper, *The Seattle Times*.

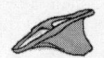

After being convicted of several offences, thirty-eight-year-old Richard Ewing from Burlington County, New Jersey decided to stop molesting young women. Good? Well, yes, of course... However, instead, he turned his attentions to having sex with cows and, in 2006, was charged again – this time with offences relating to animal cruelty.

CLOTHES MAKETH THE MAN

Shoes, socks, panties… these are common fetishes. Some people get off by wearing them, some by sniffing them and some by even stealing them. But it gets a lot weirder. Like the man who insisted he made love dressed as Napoleon and the couple who could only have sex if the man wore a frilly pink negligee and his wife donned a gas mask…

Charles Hay, thirty-seven, of Musselburgh, Scotland was jailed in 1986 after an eight-year career of assaulting women and then stealing their shoes. On one occasion, he attacked a twenty-two-year-old woman and forced her to put on a pair of her boots. He then proceeded to lick and bite the boots.

More extreme was a Paris man who struck three times in the course of three months in 1992. Each time, he broke into women's homes, stole their shoes and then forced them to watch him chew them.

IS IT IN YET?

Chuck Jones – one-time publicist for Maria Maples, the American actress and TV personality who was once married to Donald Trump – admitted having a 'physical sexual relationship' with her shoes. According to the *New York Post*, which reported the sexual harassment case brought against him, 'Some seventy of her high heels, cowboy boots, slippers and high-top Converse sneakers turned up soiled and stashed under a radiator cover in Jones' office.'

In 2008 an Australian driver was stopped by police, who suspected he was driving under the influence of drugs. Searching the car for evidence, they found eighty-one pairs of women's knickers in the glove compartment. When accused of stealing the underwear, the driver explained that they all belonged to his girlfriend. A subsequent body search for drugs revealed the man to be wearing a bright-pink lady's thong.

American James Dowdy is a serial sock sniffer, having been arrested three times for breaking into women's homes just to steal this specific item of clothing. Incidentally, the foot is among the heaviest producers of sweat in the body, generating over 0.2 imperial pints of perspiration each day.

CLOTHES MAKETH THE MAN

In September 2004 David Baron – a fifty-eight-year-old dental-equipment salesman – was discovered dead by his wife in their Gloucestershire home, wearing women's tights, a grey pleated skirt, black bra and a clear plastic apron, and hooked up to a machine pumping out nitrous oxide. The inquest heard how Mr Baron had experimented with the dental anaesthetic before but that his wife understood it was just to relax him. In a clear case of 'stating the obvious', the Cheltenham Coroner commented, 'I think this was a sexual experiment which went very badly wrong.'

Shigeo Kodama from Tokyo has the honour of being the world's greatest underwear thief. Over a six-year period, he amassed a hoard of 2,977 items of lingerie, abusing his position as a construction worker to break into women's apartments.

Thirty-one-year-old Ralph Santiago was a night security guard in Reading who made quite an impression on his first day at work in July 2008. He suffocated himself during an autoerotic accident that went wrong. His body was discovered by a colleague the following morning in a locked toilet cubicle, wearing wellington boots, a wetsuit and gas mask. During the course of the investigation, it was discovered that, the evening before he died, Mr Santiago had printed off information from the Internet explaining how arousal could be heightened by inhaling 'poppers' (legal chemicals used to stimulate a sexual high) via a gas mask. The cause of death was cardio-respiratory arrest and the coroner recorded a verdict of misadventure.

In January 2012 a Glasgow man was sentenced to community service and psychotherapy for approaching four boys and attempting to lick their trainers (as the news report states) for his 'gratification'. Police commented, 'I think it's important that he gets the help and support needed.'

In May 1990 forty-two-year-old army colonel Edward L. Modesto, of Fort Carson, Colorado was accused of wearing a wig and women's clothing and exposing himself to customers at local Laundromats. Court documents also showed that he once performed at a bar wearing a sequinned gown and lip-synching to Bette Midler songs. He was charged with conduct unbecoming of an officer.

A medical report quotes the case of a burley six-foot, four-inch police officer and his wife who had problems making love and consulted their local GP. It started when the wife said that she would only have sex if her husband wore a frilly pink negligee. Rather than be completely taken aback

CLOTHES MAKETH THE MAN

at this bizarre request, the officer agreed – as long as his wife wore a gas mask. After trying this for a while, they sought professional advice. That's when their doctor decided they needed more specialist help.

A masked gunman who held up a Berlin clothing shop in East Berlin was told that the cash register had just been emptied. Not wanting to leave empty handed, he then ordered the store manager to hand over the next best thing… all the items of women's underwear in the shop.

A twenty-eight-year-old man caught stealing young girls' panties from clothes lines in 1986 denied he'd been doing this due to some sort of fetish. He'd been taking them for two years, immersing them in a pail of water imbued with the scent of flowers and then using this water in his bath. He told police that this practice was so he would be 'respected and honoured' by other people.

Thirty-three-year-old Robert Mark Van Wagner of Port St. Lucie, Florida was arrested in April 2012 after three teenage girls reported him to police. He'd approached them with a bag of socks and asked them to put them on and run around a sports field, then return the socks to him. According to the

IS IT IN YET?

arrest report, Van Wagner told police he was acting on a 'fetish' and that he had been doing it for years in various locations.

In November 1993 staff at Perfect Sitters child-care centre in Brookfield, Milwaukee were disturbed by someone pounding heavily on the back door. To their astonishment, it was a twenty-year-old man, Lance A. Binkowski, wearing a 'onesie', sucking on a dummy and holding a teddy bear. The manager called the police but Binkowski escaped in his car, injuring three officers in the process. Binkowski later turned himself in and was charged with reckless endangerment. The police declined to comment on his attire but said he had 'his own personal reasons'.

Between August and November 2002 Ian Williams – a fifty-year-old van driver from Llandudno, north Wales – broke into the bedroom of Fiona Wellings to steal her underwear. Miss Wellings had a ground-floor room at her parent's hotel at Colwyn Bay and noticed a number of items of underwear had been going missing. Using an infrared camera and a purple thong as bait, she hoped to catch the intruder in the act. Police arrested the culprit, a Mr Williams, and, at his home, they found 472 pairs of knickers, 317 suspender belts, 115 pairs of stockings, eighty-two bras and sixty-four basques. He admitted burglary and was ordered to pay his victim £1,000 in compensation and to carry out 200 hours of unpaid community work. It

CLOTHES MAKETH THE MAN

was reported that, after his arrest, Mr Williams told police he bought the underwear at local charity shops.

In December 1995 John Pitney – a fifty-year-old postal clerk from Denver – arrived at work wearing a dress and exhibiting what co-workers described as 'bizarre behaviour'. He was put on administrative leave and ordered out of the building. However, he later returned, having augmented his outfit with a gorilla mask and 'a strap-on sexual device' and was arrested.

In March 1994 forty-eight-year-old David W. Shaw – Superintendent of Schools in Hampden, New York state – was arrested for drunk driving. As if that wasn't a bad enough example to set students, in his arrest photo Shaw is wearing men's trousers but blue eye shadow, a gold lamé blouse, a string of black beads and what was described as a 'ladies' undergarment'. Shaw blamed the incident on alcohol, which he said also caused him to mistake an adult bookstore for a convenience store when he needed to buy cigarettes.

Police in Madison, Wisconsin failed to catch a man reported to be wearing just a nappy and a garter belt, who would chase women in the street, begging them to spank him.

IS IT IN YET?

Tokyo police charged Yoichi Ishihara, twenty-nine, with breaking into 150 school locker rooms to steal items of clothing. They found 1,200 pairs of schoolgirls' panties in his apartment. He explained that he had started taking the underwear as a hobby.

In August 2004 numerous Delaware motorists reported that a man was wandering along the hard shoulder of I-95. They weren't unduly worried about his safety; their main concern was with what he was wearing… or rather wasn't wearing. The man was completely naked apart from panties and a bra, which he wore on his head.

In 2008 Torao Fukuda was caught and arrested for stealing American-football uniforms from college locker rooms. He cited his love of sweat as his defence.

A woman named only as Elly was taken aback on her wedding night after her husband Oscar came to bed dressed in the full regalia of Napoleon Bonaparte. She reluctantly allowed him to have sex with her on the condition that he removed his thigh-high boots and hat – but then decided she'd had enough of being chafed by the uniform and the medals and demanded he take everything off. Oscar not only refused but also filed for divorce.

CLOTHES MAKETH THE MAN

In August 2003 a man, thought to be in his forties, exposed himself to two women in Chelmsford, Essex. The witnesses said he was wearing a pink lycra bikini and, after exposing himself, did a dance in front of them and then asked if he could kiss their feet. PC Tim Neate commented, 'The women were not harmed but we are concerned about this man's strange behaviour.'

In January 1992 a thirty-one-year-old man turned himself in to police in Anchorage, Alaska, claiming to be the fugitive known as 'Dr Diaper'. Posing as a doctor, he'd hire childminders to look after one of his patients, 'Tommy', who, according to the doctor, was an adult with the mental age of an eighteen-month-old. After making arrangements, the doctor said he would send Tommy over to them. The person who turned up, however, was actually the so-called doctor, naked apart from a giant nappy. He would then defecate in the nappy in front of them and, if he had time, masturbate too.

In a similar incident, a twenty-five-year-old man from Holladay in Utah would show up at day-care centres in the Salt Lake City area wearing baby clothes and a nappy, with the excuse that he was on a fraternity pledge. When inside the centre, he would often keep his hand inside his nappy, complaining to staff that it was 'too tight.' He was eventually arrested and charged with perversion and trespassing.

IS IT IN YET?

Just what is it about grown men and nappies? An unidentified man in his twenties wearing just a T-shirt and a nappy went into a convenience store in York, Pennsylvania and bought a can of squirty cream. The clerk commented that, after paying for the cream, the customer shook the can and sprayed it into a tube that was poking out of his nappy. He then left and drove off in a sports car. Police were baffled by the man's behaviour and commented that it was the third incident of its kind they could remember.

Since being demobbed after the Second World War a German army officer suffered from impotence, but discovered that he could overcome this condition by running a German flag up a flagpole in his garden (just outside Cologne), and donning his uniform just before he had sex. A newspaper report stated that his wife was grateful for his newfound lease of life in the bedroom but had developed a skin infection from his medals.

A policewoman visiting a ladies' toilet in Tring, Hertfordshire discovered a man wearing only a black corset. According to the local paper, when questioned, the man said that 'he was just being sociable.'

PLANES, TRAINS AND AUTOMOBILES

Tales of sex in, on and with cars, like the man who's had over a thousand lovers – only one with two legs; the rest all had four wheels. Plus deviant acts involving other modes of transport, like the man caught having sex with his bicycle, or the farmer who used his tractor in his bizarre sex games...

Therapists at London's Institute of Psychiatry reported on a twenty-year-old patient known as George. George sought their help after he found he was only able to become aroused when sitting in the family car – an Austin Metro – or by squatting behind it with the engine running.

In October 2006 two cleaners at the Aberley House Hostel in Ayr, south-west Scotland tried to get into the room of guest

IS IT IN YET?

Robert Stewart. After knocking several times and getting no reply, they opened the door using a master key, only to see fifty-one-year-old Mr Roberts naked from the waist down, thrusting his hips back and forth and simulating sex with a bicycle. Both witnesses were extremely shocked and notified the hotel manager, who, in turn, alerted the police.

Mr Stewart was placed on the sex offenders' register and put on probation for three years.

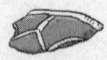

Canadian Sandy Wong was arrested in 2007 at Edmonton's Home and Garden Show, for masturbating next to a display of classic cars. Two years earlier, he'd been arrested for rubbing sexually against a Mini Cooper.

Having sex in a car can be exciting but can also have tragic consequences, as Romanian first-division football player Mario Bugeanu and his girlfriend Mirela Iancu discovered to their cost in 1999. Their mistake was that Mario left the car in his garage with the engine running. The couple died from carbon-monoxide poisoning and were discovered by the player's father the next day.

PLANES, TRAINS AND AUTOMOBILES

A *ménage à trois* ended in A&E when a man and two girls attempted to have sex in a parked car in the city of Wenzhou, China in June 2014. Soon after the threesome began, the man, Chung Yeh, accidentally kicked the handbrake off and the car started to roll downhill before violently crashing into a tree. Although Yeh was uninjured and managed to climb out to raise the alarm, it took two dozen firemen to cut the women free from the vehicle, one of whom had broken both her legs.

Over the last forty-five years, sixty-two-year-old Edward Smith from Washington State has had sex with over a thousand lovers but only one has been a person; the rest have all been cars. A self-confessed 'mechaphile' (someone sexually attracted to machines), Smith first became attracted to cars in his teens. At his peak, he was having sex with one a week. These days, though, he's in a committed relationship with his 1969 Volkswagen Beetle, which he calls Vanilla. In a newspaper interview, Smith said, 'When I hold Vanilla in my arms, there's a powerful energy that comes from her. I would say it is extremely satisfying but at times a little melancholy because I know she cannot talk to me. But overall, I know she feels what I feel and it's intense.'

Despite being in a long-term relationship with the Beetle, Smith did admit that sometimes he's tempted to stray, saying, 'I will not deny that I look at other cars on TV or at shows and still get those old impulses and desires – but those were the early days. Now I want to settle down with Vanilla.'

IS IT IN YET?

In May 2009 a drunk American couple were arrested after police spotted them having sex in their car. Local police in Ohio reported that Danica Wallace, twenty-four, and lover Jeremy Welch, twenty-nine, pulled off the roadway to have sex in the Ford Taurus that she was driving. When police approached the vehicle, they found Welch in the front passenger seat. Astride him was Wallace, naked from the waist down. Oh, yes... in the back, looking on, were her children, aged just four and twenty-two months. Welch explained his actions by telling the police, 'We got horny and just wanted to fuck.'

Canadian Terence Mikoch, thirty-one, was arrested when the United Airlines plane on which he was travelling landed at Los Angeles in 1987. The reason? He'd crept up behind one of the stewardesses who was preparing coffee in the galley and fondled her breasts, thighs and buttocks. She turned around and hit him with the coffee pot – and he responded by dropping his trousers and exposing himself. The reason he gave for his actions was that he believed he was on board a spaceship bound for another world and that the stewardess was merely an android. Mikoch was ordered by the Los Angeles court to seek psychiatric help.

In July 2009 a train driver was seen by another crew member performing a sex act at the controls of a high-speed London-

PLANES, TRAINS AND AUTOMOBILES

to-Glasgow Virgin train, with a pornographic magazine on his lap. The incident was reported to senior managers when the train arrived in Scotland and the driver was suspended pending a disciplinary investigation. News reports at the time took great satisfaction in reporting that the driver had been 'pulled from duty'.

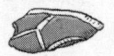

In 1999, in the town of Okeechobee in Florida, two men came across a Honda SUV idling with no one in it and then noticed someone's feet protruding from underneath it. On further investigation, they discovered that the feet belonged to their friend Bryan Loudermilk, who was lying in a ditch with one of the car's tyres parked on his stomach. A news report of the incident quotes them as asking what he was doing and Loudermilk replying that he couldn't feel his legs. One of the friends then asked if he wanted the car moved off him, to which his friend said, 'Yes.' As they carefully moved the car, they noticed that this was no bizarre accident. The car's tyre had been resting on a board and this was on top of a pillow on Loudermilk's chest.

A medical report stated that, as soon as the pressure was relieved, lactic acid and other toxins flooded from his bloodless legs through the rest of his circulatory system, poisoning his body and initiating shock. The emergency services were called but Loudermilk died on the way to hospital. In the days that followed, police pieced together a startling story that briefly became national news. Loudermilk was into the sexual fetishes of 'trampling', where he was aroused by being stepped on by women, particularly his 200-lb wife. When he lay down under his SUV that afternoon, police believe he was taking his fetish to the extreme. One question remains unanswered: Police still have no idea who helped Loudermilk with his obsession by parking his car on top of him.

A couple who decided to have sex in the back of their car parked it by the River Enns, near the city of Graz in Austria. In the height of passion, they failed to realise that the vehicle was slowly creeping forward. The handbrake hadn't been applied properly and the energetic movement in the car caused it to slip down an embankment into the cold waters, where it sank. The couple managed to escape and swim, unharmed (but completely naked), to the riverbank.

When a waitress and a female passenger on board a busy Glasgow ScotRail service from Dundee to Perth rebuffed the advances of twenty-five-year-old Andrew Davidson, he turned his attentions to the next best thing – the drinks trolley. The incident took place in July 2013 and Perth Sheriff's Court heard how Davidson was seen thrusting himself against the trolley saying, 'I want to kiss you, I want to fuck you.' According to *STV News*, Davidson's solicitor told the court his client had 'gone crazy after taking a legal high.' Ahead of his sentencing, Davidson had been placed on the Sex Offenders Register but was removed after the

PLANES, TRAINS AND AUTOMOBILES

Sheriff said he did not consider the sexual element of the case to be 'significant'.

In September 1992 Maria Ramos and Darryl Washington were injured at New York's Bowery subway station when a train ran over them while they had sex on a mattress they'd thrown on to the tracks. Miraculously, neither of them was seriously hurt. She'd escaped with cuts and bruises, while he suffered a broken leg and fractured vertebra. Recovering at Bellevue Hospital, Washington told reporters, 'I started kissing her. I closed my eyes, and the next thing I knew, something went "BANG!" It was a very big bang.' A shaken Ramos told detectives, 'Usually, no trains run on that track.'

In November 2012 Callum Ward from Barnstaple in Devon was spotted by police thrusting himself against an ambulance and then simulating a sex act on its bonnet. Described as being 'in relatively high spirits' while the offences took place, Ward was found guilty of being drunk and disorderly and in possession of Class B drugs, and was sentenced to a community order and a £60 fine. Barnstaple Magistrates Court was told that, earlier that day, Ward was seen setting fire to a peanut packet inside a phone box.

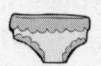

IS IT IN YET?

Fearing a terrorist incident in July 2014, the NYPD harbour unit were on high alert when they were called to investigate a fishing boat that had crashed into runway approach lights that extend into New York harbour from the city's La Guardia Airport. Arriving at the scene, it took the police thirty minutes to establish that there was no security risk. The boat had crashed and impaled itself on a lighting stanchion after the boat's owner – fifty-one-year-old James Gallo – and passengers James Benenato and Mary Ann Belson – both sixty – were all below deck enjoying a three-way sex session. The *New York Post* reported, 'There's a moral here: If you're feeling amorous aboard a boat, drop your anchor before you drop your pants.'

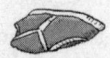

Romanian couple Robert Filip and Andrea Popescu were getting very amorous in their car; she was performing oral sex on her naked boyfriend. The only problem was that he was driving at the time. The pleasure was so intense that Robert swerved off the road and crashed into a parked car. Even this didn't distract Andrea, who continued to pleasure her boyfriend without missing a stroke.

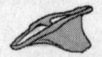

When indulging in a solo sexual act, it's good to think about what would happen if anything should go wrong and you were discovered by a loved one. One sixty-two-year-old American man didn't heed this advice so, when his wife came across his body, she was understandably shocked. She found him trapped under the front scoop of his tractor, naked apart from a pair of women's red stilettos and stockings, and with duct tape wrapped around his ankles. His clothing was found folded neatly nearby, next to a fishing-tackle box containing women's jewellery and two packets of tights. Investigators concluded that the victim's method of sexual self-stimulation was to suspend himself upside down from the tractor while he cross-dressed, using ropes to control the raising and lowering of the scoop. For some reason the scoop had dropped, coming to rest on his back and pinning him to the ground. The cause of death was positional asphyxiation by chest compression.

Greg Penser and Melissa De Carli of Waterbury, Connecticut were in their parked car getting very amorous when a truck driven by Victor Reynolds crashed into them. They claim the shock of the accident caused Greg to ejaculate and they sued the truck driver for $1 million for causing Melissa to become pregnant. Greg commented, 'I don't wear protection because Melissa doesn't like it, so I'm always very careful – but then the truck hit us I couldn't help myself.' The outcome of their legal action is unknown.

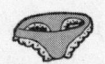

IS IT IN YET?

In February 2009 witnesses called police when they saw a man seated in his car at a supermarket kissing two inflatable sex dolls. Officers arrived at the Cape Coral, Florida location to find a crowd of people gathered around the car, shouting and pointing at fifty-one-year-old George Bartusek, who was not wearing any underwear. He was arrested on charges of trespassing and disturbing the peace after witnesses gave statements alleging that they had seen him performing 'simulated sexual activity' with the dolls.

According to police, on his arrest, Bartusek told officers that he had gone to the store to buy clothes for the two dolls.

In September 2014 a fifty-six-year-old man wearing eye shadow and lipstick was arrested by police as he masturbated in his car near a truck stop in Syracus, New York. He was reported by several truck drivers and charged with public lewdness. His name? Calvin E. Wank.

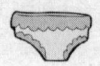

Rather than have sex in his car in a deserted spot, which might be an obvious location, Florian Neuz and his mistress Steffi Klose decided to throw caution to the wind and, instead, have sex in the boot while parked on the hard shoulder of the busy A7 autobahn. Unfortunately, the boot lid slammed shut on them and they were forced to embarrassingly call the police from Steffi's mobile phone.

PLANES, TRAINS AND AUTOMOBILES

Police arriving at the scene of a car crash in Ronda, Spain found the slightly injured drivers in one car naked. A police officer told reporters afterwards, 'The man claimed the collision stripped him but we don't believe him.'

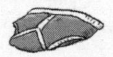

In 2006 a Danish man who was accused of flashing came up with a rather novel excuse for why he'd exposed himself on public transport. He unsuccessfully tried to convince the Oslo court that a bee had flown into his underpants and that the only way he could get it out was to open his fly and wave his penis about to try and encourage the angry insect to leave.

In April 2012 Michael Galvin came up with an equally preposterous excuse for exposing himself to a fellow passenger on the B-Line trolley car in Boston. Rather than being intimidated or upset by his behaviour, the unnamed passenger restrained him until police arrived to arrest him. Galvin was charged with 'open and gross lewdness' but told police that the trolley was really crowded and that the 'jostling' caused his shorts to fall off and that he was unaware he was exposed.

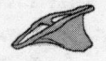

A man and his girlfriend were having sex in the back seat of a small sports car in London's Regent's Park when the man suddenly and painfully slipped a disc and couldn't move. What's more, he weighed 200 lbs, so the woman was trapped beneath him. Realising they needed to be rescued, she managed to honk the horn with one of her feet, which soon alerted a small crowd and, eventually, firemen and cutting gear. The roof of the car was removed and the man lifted out and taken to hospital. The woman was all right, apart from worrying about how she'd explain to her husband what had happened to his prized car.

In May 1992 a thirty-seven-year-old Minneapolis man was charged with indecent exposure after several keen-eyed witnesses reported him driving his car naked from the waist down. After a long chase that involved several collisions with other vehicles, police managed to apprehend the man. As the witnesses had described, he *was* naked from the waist down… apart from four $1 bills stuck to his penis. Police later said that they had stopped him several time before, naked but with higher-denomination notes attached.

Police called to the scene of a car crash in the Abruzzo region of southern Italy in May 2000 were surprised to see that the two bodies in the wreckage (a couple, known only as Germano and Franciska) were completely naked and apparently having sex when the driver lost control on a bend. It's common for Italian youngsters to have sex in their car when parents frown on relations before marriage, but why this couple were doing it at eighty miles an hour remains a mystery.

PLANES, TRAINS AND AUTOMOBILES

A forty-year-old airline pilot got his kicks by being dragged behind his car, until the fateful day when he chained himself to his VW and set the steering wheel and accelerator so it would just drive around in circles in a deserted parking lot. During the process, the chains got tangled and he was crushed to death against his own car.

SERIOUS SHORTCOMINGS

Some men are content with their lack of endowment, or have at least come to terms with their limitations. Others, however, have gone further and have embraced their small penises (not literally) in poetry, pageants and parties…

Charged with flashing, a Texan man claimed mistaken identity, saying that his penis was so small that no woman would have been able to spot it. The court in Houston upheld his conviction, despite conceding that his penis was only 2.8 inches long.

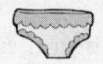

Similarly, when forty-one-year-old Doug Neece from Davenport, Iowa appeared in court on indecent-exposure charges in February 2004, his wife Sheila acted as a defence witness – although he probably wished she hadn't. Sheila told the jury that Doug wasn't well-endowed enough to be seen from any distance and that there was no way that he could be guilty of flashing at a postwoman. Despite her damning evidence, Doug was jailed.

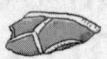

In August 2002, a group of male friends from Antipolo City in the Philippines went out drinking and soon the subject got round to penis size… and a challenge to see who had the biggest. When it was Arnel Orbeta's time, he unzipped to present his penis, which wasn't that impressive. His pal Eduardo Cristomar started laughing, so Arnel reacted in the way any affronted man would (wouldn't they?) – he shot Eduardo six times in the head and groin.

Ernest Hemingway's small penis was once described as being 'the size of a .30-30 rifle shell.' That's a maximum size of 12.9 mm wide x 52 mm long.

June 2014 saw what has been described as 'The city's least visually impressive pageant': The Smallest Penis in Brooklyn Pageant. The second time this event had been held saw a host of contestants displaying their modest members in the King's County Bar. The eventual winner was New Delhi

SERIOUS SHORTCOMINGS

native Raj Kumar, a twenty-eight-year-old who works in digital advertising. As well as the honour, he received a glitter encrusted, penis-spired crown. Reports of the event stated that Kumar seemed genuinely touched at the turnout and oddly proud of his new title.

In case you're wondering, the title was won purely on appearance… no rulers were used.

British urologists Kevan Wylie and Ian Eardley's comprehensive review of more than fifty studies into Small Penis Syndrome revealed (unsurprisingly) that men have more sexual confidence if they have a large penis.

London-based author and poet Ant Smith admits he has a small penis and campaigns to abolish penis-size anxiety. To help deal with the shame and stigma that surrounds small tackle, he wrote the poem 'Shorty', which he first performed at a 'Sing for Your Supper' open-mic night. Smith said, 'Before performing this poem, I ask the audience if they're ready for some truth. Four minutes of powerful punishing truth. I then launch into the opening line, declaring my diminutive self:

"I have a tiny cock
Like a crooked little finger.
Everybody else's dick
Is inevitably bigger."'

IS IT IN YET?

Smith also commented, 'Once I'd written the first draft of "Shorty", I knew I had to perform it. Otherwise, I'd be a hypocrite.'

(In case you're interested, it's four inches long.)

Napoleon Bonaparte's physician, Francesco Autommarchi, removed the late emperor's penis while conducting his autopsy. His post-mortem described the member as 'very small' and its length was recorded at just 1.5 inches. Since then, the penis has been in the hands of collectors across the world and, at the time of writing, resides in New Jersey, in the home of Evan Lattimer, whose father – a renowned urologist – bought it at a Paris auction for $3,000. Mr Lattimer has only allowed ten people to view the withered relic, which is known in the family as 'Napoleon's item'.

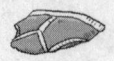

According to *The Atlas of Human Sex Anatomy*, the normal length of a soft penis ranges from 8.4–10.5 cm (3.3–4.13 in), with an erection adding about 30 per cent to the size. Sexologist Alfred Kinsey reported than 90 per cent of men have an average-sized penis.

The sexologist recorded a patient whose penis was only 2.5 cm (1 in) when erect. In some medical conditions, where the penis fails to develop properly, an erect penis may not exceed 1 cm (0.4 in) in length. These are called, appropriately enough, micropenises.

SERIOUS SHORTCOMINGS

If you're worried about the size of your manhood, share a thought for the poor gorilla that has the smallest penis-to-body-size ratio of any mammal. Although an adult male can weigh up to 280 kg (617 lbs), it only has an erection of about 5 cm.

Britain's Big Small Penis Party took place in March of this year. While well-endowed men were not barred from attending, the admission fee was charged by the inch. Performers at the event included comedians, poets, folk musicians and rappers but the organisers were clear to point out that this wasn't a 'pity party' but a celebration of good things coming in small packages, stating, 'It's an open invite to everybody, male or female. We've all been touched by a small penis in our lifetime; now's the time to give something back.'

TAKEN FOR A RIDE

It's amazing how gullible people can be… from the optician who convinced his patients that they needed to be naked while he prescribed contact lenses, to the man who persuaded women that he had a spaceship and that, to overcome space sickness before he took them for a spin, they first needed to have sex with him. There's one born every minute…

James Marriner – a police sergeant from Queensland, Australia – approached a right-wing religious group called the Christian Brethren and said he needed their help to work undercover and smash a local paedophile ring. Only too pleased to assist the forces of law and order, the group was then astonished to learn that they had to cut off their pubic hair and take photos of themselves naked; Marriner convinced them that these actions were necessary before they became police informants.

IS IT IN YET?

This went on for eighteen years, after which time the group found out there was no paedophile ring and that Marriner had requested and received the pubic hair and photographs for his own sexual gratification. He was jailed for five years in October 2003. At the trial, Judge Manus Boyce commented, 'There is overwhelming evidence that you are a very devious pervert.'

Texas gynaecologist Dr William Clark tricked a woman into taking part in a bogus pain-research project in 1987. This involved him taking her blood pressure while he spanked her.

He lost his licence.

A Chinese acupuncturist from Reading was accused of fondling his assistant's breasts in 1989. He claimed he was just searching for an acupuncture point called the *jing jong*.

A nineteen-year-old man in Atlanta, Georgia would masquerade as a top music-video producer just so he could attract girls. When they fell for his promise of a lucrative recording career and pop stardom, he revealed that all he really wanted them to do was bite his belly button.

TAKEN FOR A RIDE

Householders in Bad Urach in Germany were only too pleased to help the smartly-dressed middle-aged man who called at their home saying that his car had broken down and that he needed to use their phone. However, they became suspicious when he would stay on the line for fifteen minutes, getting more and more flustered, obviously excited about something more than trying to sort out a breakdown vehicle. It turned out that he'd been calling premium-rate sex lines.

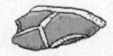

A fifty-year-old chartered accountant spent three hours on the phone to a nursing home in Eastbourne, posing as someone investigating a series of thefts by cleaning staff. He managed to persuade a head nurse to conduct an intimate body search of a young woman cleaner while he was on the phone, which culminated, strangely, in the nurse cutting three inches from the cleaner's hair. The call was traced to the man's home in Harlow, Essex and he admitted making hundreds of similar calls and having a fixation about hair. Despite the distance involved, he was charged with assault.

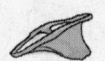

A Canberra man had a liaison with a prostitute in October 2010 and booked her for a second session at a cost of $800. On this occasion, after they had sex, he handed her a bulky sealed envelope, telling her not to check for the money as it would spoil any romance — and that he needed her to trust him. He left and you can guess the outcome: when she opened the envelope, there was no money, just a folded-up paper bag.

An immigration official at Toronto's Pearson International Airport was suspended after ordering visitors to take their shoes and socks off so he could photograph their feet, telling them that this was 'official policy.' The airport acknowledged that, following complaints, the agent had been counselled for this behaviour on four previous occasions.

Before prescribing contact lenses, a Belgian optician from Brasschaat would ask his patients to strip naked and dance around his consulting room while he played the accordion. He appeared in court in March 1995 but was acquitted of any wrongdoing after his lawyer successfully argued that he had qualified in England, where he believed this behaviour was commonplace.

In 1999 a thief successfully duped a number of women in Osaka, Japan by telling them there had been a virulent outbreak of the highly infectious e coli 0157:H7 bacteria in the city and that the way to protect themselves was to hand him their knickers.

TAKEN FOR A RIDE

Manfred Kah was a twenty-nine-year-old bank manager from Cologne in Germany, who posed as a Dr Bender. He would call random women up all over the country and tell them he was treating a relative of theirs with a malignant disease and that he needed to make sure they weren't carrying the virus. The special test apparently involved him having sex with them until they reached orgasm. He explained that he had to do this a few times 'just to make sure of the diagnosis.' Later, he would call them and tell them the test was, thankfully, negative.

Until he was eventually arrested, Dr Bender had sex with at least 160 gullible women.

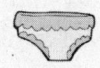

Tax inspector Stephen Davidson, forty-two, posed as film producer in search of a girl who could give the 'perfect scream'. He kept this pretence up for a six-year period until 1981, luring hundreds of girls from New York universities for auditions. In his studio, they were told they needed to be topless and were given a red miniskirt and a straw boater to wear. Davidson would then spank them and judge the quality of their scream. The girls really believed they'd get a film contract; they had no idea Davidson was only taking the opportunity to secretly photograph the spankings, which were then sold to porno mags.

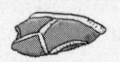

IS IT IN YET?

In 2011 Kevin Gausepohl – a thirty-four-year-old music teacher from Tacoma, Washington – was convicted of communicating with a minor for immoral purposes. He'd told a seventeen-year-old student that she would sing better if she was naked, telling her he was conducting a study on how sexual arousal affects vocal ranges. The girl stripped and touched herself on a couple of occasions before getting suspicious. Gausepohl is said to have pitched his 'getting naked will improve your singing' idea to several students.

Nicole Lindsay – a twenty-four-year-old single mother from Glasgow – was stunned to discover that her boyfriend was actually a twenty-six-year-old woman and former lesbian sex offender, Samantha Brooks, who went by the name of Lee. Intimate details of the case were widely reported, including how Samantha claimed she'd had scarring on her torso where a previous lover had burned her, which is why she had to wear tight bandages around her chest, and how she made excuses for not showing her genitals by claiming she had testicular cancer. The couple, however, had regular sex over a number of years and police found in her possession a fake penis made from the wooden centre of a toilet-roll holder, padded out with bandages and overlaid with four condoms.

Samantha/Lee maintained this charade for a number of years, although Nicole said that one of her uncles was suspicious, saying that Lee didn't have an Adam's apple and commenting that his handshake wasn't 'manly'. The couple first met in 2006 but, in 2011, Brooks was charged with obtaining sex by deception from Nicole and a former friend but the case collapsed when the friend withdrew her co-operation from prosecutors. Afterwards, Nicole told the press, 'I can see areas where maybe she was trying to be very careful but, in other ways, she was completely brazen and totally confident she had me a hundred per cent fooled. And she was right.'

Between 2003 and 2006 Roland Rudman of Torquay secretly filmed the legs and feet of over a hundred unsuspecting women. His ploy was more ingenious. He'd pretend that his car had broken down and he'd ask women in skirts to help him. All they had to do was sit in the driver's seat and rev the engine while he made adjustments under the bonnet. What they didn't know was that he'd installed a miniature camera in the footwell to film their legs. One of his victims discovered what was happening but, due to a technically in the case, Rudman was spared jail. However, he did receive a ten-year ASBO, banning him for approaching any women with the aim of filming them.

In 2006 an unnamed Solihull student started receiving threatening text messages and phone calls from an Asian male who said he would kidnap her and force her to convert to Islam. She confided in her friend, Harvinder Singh

IS IT IN YET?

Jheeta, who gallantly said he'd go to the police and make the complaint on her behalf and sort it out. The student then started receiving texts, supposedly from police officers in charge of the investigation, including one telling her to have sex with Jheeta, which she did on several occasions. Jheeta, at first, denied that it was him behind the texts but then admitted it, adding that he 'probably needed his head testing.'

Jheeta's defence lawyer described him as a 'rather pathetic young man' and he pleaded guilty at his trial in September 2006 to two charges of procuring a young woman to have intercourse with him by false pretences. He was jailed for eight years.

In 2003 a young woman collapsed in a Leicester bar and paramedics were called. In the meantime, one of the other drinkers rushed to help, saying he was a qualified first-aider. Onlookers became suspicious, however, when he tested her pulse by squeezing her breasts. He was arrested when the real first-aiders arrived.

Bulgarian Georgio Barrsan, fifty-six, almost cleared out his bank account and pawned his wedding ring in order to enjoy an ultimate night of debauchery. He used the money to buy a large supply of black-market Viagra and the services of two hookers. He woke up the next morning with no recollection of endless wild sex – just a sore head and the realisation that his wallet and all his money had been stolen. The tablets he'd bought had been sleeping pills.

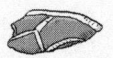

A man in his late twenties conned his library in Midwest City, Oklahoma into lending him a room where he could conduct a series of job interviews for a secretarial post for a local civic organisation. Thirteen women applied and were interviewed and discovered they had to undergo what he called the 'Johnson Stress Test'. This involved them being blindfolded and taking dictation in three positions: standing up with their feet wide apart, sitting on a desk and bending over the desk. While they were blindfolded, he was looking up their dresses. Police revealed his MO when they discovered he'd pulled the same stunt at other city libraries.

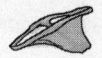

Barry Briskman – a fifty-seven-year-old from Los Angeles – would seduce women by claiming he came from the planet Cablell and promising them a ride in his spaceship. Anyone gullible enough to fall for that line would then be told that, to overcome space sickness, they'd have to have sex with him. After seducing a number of underage women in this way, he was arrested and jailed for twenty years.

IS IT IN YET?

Raymond Mitchell III, forty-five, of Tennessee would call women at random, pretending he was their boyfriend and telling them he wanted to meet for sex… but that they'd need to be blindfolded. Prosecutors said that most of the hundreds of women that Mitchell rang hung up on him but, of the thirty who reported him to the police, eight had actually been tricked into sex. One woman admitted that she'd had sex with him twice a week for two months until the day her blindfold slipped and she found out it wasn't her actual boyfriend.

A thirty-eight-year-old man was approached by a man in a Salt Lake City bar asking for a lift home. He told police that, during the journey, they started talking about sex and then stopped the car so they could fondle each other. During the groping, the stranger grabbed the driver's $300 watch and ran off. The victim told police that he didn't get a good look at the thief's face but that he 'would be able to identify him by the feel of his genitals.'

A Hong Kong Court convicted a former police officer of 'unlawful sex acts by false pretences' when he posed as a doctor and told a woman that having sex with him was the only way she could prevent unscrupulous doctors from cutting off her husband's penis. She believed him.

TAKEN FOR A RIDE

A man in Oakland, California masquerading as a doctor told recently arrived immigrants that they carried a rare virus and that, in order to avoid deportation, they had to receive a special serum. This serum could only be released into their bodies by sexual intercourse.

A doctor in Bay City, Texas persuaded a woman to participate in a crucial 'Pain Research Study' and the chance to earn $2,500 if he could spank her. She agreed and submitted to sixteen spanking sessions, some lasting up to ninety minutes, over a two-month period. She complained when he failed to pay her and that's when the Texan authorities discovered that, not only did the research project not exist but the doctor had been suspended by the Louisiana state medical board for pulling the same stunt.

A student who'd just had a tanning session at the Consol Centre in Cardiff was about to leave when she was called back by Peter Bush, forty-nine, who said he was a sun-bed engineer and needed her to lie down in one of the cubicles while he tested the equipment. She did what he said but, instead of carrying out his calibrations, Mr Bush exposed himself. According to reports, the student ran out when she saw him committing a sex act. Serial flasher Bush pleaded guilty to indecent exposure at Cardiff Crown Court. His defence lawyer claimed he committed offences on the spur of

IS IT IN YET?

the moment 'while under stress.' Bush was given a three-year community sentence with attendance on a Sex Offenders' Treatment programme.

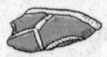

A St Louis police officer was accused of stopping at least ten women for minor traffic violations. The women reported that he would tell them to sit in the back seat of his car and remove their shoes, explaining that shoes were a potential hiding place for drugs. He would then fondle or tickle their feet – or merely stare at them.

Thirty-six-year-old Roy McCarthy was caught by police after a series of incidents whereby he'd 'accidentally' drop bottles of wine on the feet of grocery-store workers in Clayton, Missouri and then rub their toes, telling them he was a doctor. Store officials became suspicious after staff started reporting a spate of wine-bottle-related foot injuries.

MISCELLANEOUS

Why 'Miscellaneous'? Well, sometimes there's no natural home for unnatural acts. Like the man who broke into women's apartments and rearranged their shoes, the driving instructor who kept a twelve-inch carrot down his trousers and the ninety-one-year-old woman who ordered a statuette of the Virgin Mary and who, instead, received a nine-inch dildo...

Janitor Marcelino Castro of California claimed that two 'large Samoans' had held him down at work and inserted a huge dildo up his rectum. Police took the claim very seriously but, after lengthy investigations to track the offenders down, discovered that the janitor had made the story up to conceal his love of anal pleasures. He was fined the equivalent of £28,000 for wasting police time.

IS IT IN YET?

In November 2007 a thirty-five-year-old homeless man, James Macnair, was arrested for breaking into a church in Valley Cottage, New York State but, to the surprise of police officers, it wasn't to steal the collection box; it was to use the phone at the Elim Alliance Church to call a sex hotline. Macnair was charged with two counts of burglary, possession of a burglar's tools and petty larceny. When arrested, he told police that he'd broken into the church the previous week for the same purpose.

Ninety-one-year-old Adelaide Douglas of Queensland, Australia got quite a shock when she opened a package containing what she thought was a statuette of the Virgin Mary from AVA Enterprises. The box actually contained a nine-inch dildo and a sex manual. A spokesman for the company explained that they deal in both religious trinkets and sex aids and that, unfortunately, mix-ups sometimes occurred.

Italian physics student Lino Missio was granted a patent in 1994 for his musical condom. Designed to alert the user in case of an accident, the condom plays Beethoven when it splits.

MISCELLANEOUS

Mary Verdev, seventy-three, sued a Milwaukee church for $90,000 after an electronic bingo scoreboard fell on her head and changed her personality. She claimed that, after the accident, she became attracted to women and had spontaneous orgasms.

Driving instructor Stephen Cooney, fifty-one, from Cleveland had an unusual way of encouraging one of his female students. He grabbed the woman's hand and placed it on his groin so she could feel his twelve-inch penis. Except it wasn't his penis. It was a carrot. The unnamed victim told Teesside Crown Court, 'He said, "You've got me so excited." He said it was because my driving was so good. I was shocked; disgusted. I thought I had got hold of an erection. Then he pulled the carrot out from down his flies, where it must have been throughout my lesson.'

Prosecutor Rod Hunt said, 'When you go to a driving instructor, you may expect he would carry a copy of the Highway Code. You would not expect him to drive around with a twelve-inch carrot down his trousers, pretending he had an erection.'

Cooney was jailed for eighteen months.

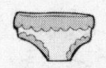

IS IT IN YET?

According to the *New York Daily News*, New York City Correction Department doctor Jerzy Gajewski was put on trial for fondling a woman in a subway station in 1992 but, before a verdict could be reached, he allegedly fondled the court stenographer.

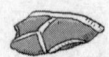

To make sure their lovers were really turned on in the bedroom, women in Ancient China often embroidered their underwear with pornographic scenes.

Some types of codpiece, which were popular with men eager to show off their sexual attributes in the fifteenth to seventeenth centuries, contained secret pockets in which the wearer would keep small pieces of fruit in order to tempt women.

In the 1980s a number of 'no knickers' tea and coffee shops opened in Tokyo, with waitresses wearing very skimpy miniskirts in order to titillate customers.

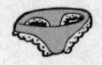

MISCELLANEOUS

In October 2002 a Mr Rosaire Roy of Prince Albert, Saskatchewan was sentenced to a year in prison for hiring someone to rob his store. His motive, however, was not to collect insurance money but to fulfil a sexual fantasy. He had arranged for the thief to force him and an unsuspecting female friend who was in the store at the time to undress because he'd always dreamed of being tied up naked with her.

In March 1997 *The Economist* reported that, when their company had insufficient cash to pay their wages, workers at the Akhtuba factory in Volgograd were paid, instead, in rubber dildos. Unfortunately, workers who tried to sell their dildos to local sex shops were very disappointed; the market had long since moved on to electric vibrators and inert dildos were unsalable.

Male nurse Brian Mallon was supposed to be supervising three mentally handicapped swimmers. Instead, he was having sex in the pool with a woman he'd just met moments earlier. Mallon told authorities that the swimmers weren't at any risk because he had his eye on them the whole time. 'Besides,' he argued, 'the act only took half a minute.'

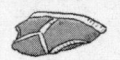

IS IT IN YET?

Twenty-four-year-old Steve Danos from Baton Rouge, Louisiana became known as the Serial Snuggler. He was eventually caught in March 2003 after entering the apartments of twelve young women through unlocked doors or windows but, rather than assault them, he would snuggle next to them when they slept and occasionally folded their laundry or arranged their shoes. He was sentenced to five years' probation and 200 hours of community service.

Jose Barbosa broke into several shops in Manila, The Philippines in 1996 but, since he never actually stole anything, could only be arrested for breaking and entering. Once inside the shops, he used their phones to call sex lines. One store was billed $20,000 in a single month.

In order to look sexy, fashionable Japanese women used to paint their teeth black, while, to achieve the same effect, women in Greenland would paint their faces blue and yellow.

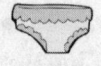

The Cincinnati Enquirer reported a story in 2008 that involved a girl falling asleep during sex. Her partner was more than disappointed by this reflection on his performance. To show his displeasure, he set fire to her car.

MISCELLANEOUS

You're never too old to have a perversion, as eighty-five-year-old Fred Burton of Horndean, Hampshire demonstrated. In 2004 he was discovered dead in his home with string tied around his genitals, having choked to death on a rubber bathing cap.

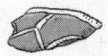

In 1993, after police raided the A1 Massage Studio in Oregon, they discovered that it offered a masturbation service offered by two sisters. They were aged seventy and seventy-three.

Suspecting his wife Catherine of infidelity, Russian czar Peter the Great had her suspected lover, William Mons, killed and his head pickled in alcohol and placed in her bedroom.

Similarly, when King John of England suspected his wife Isabella of Angouleme of being unfaithful, he had her lover hanged and he suspended his corpse above her bed.

Leszek Szwerowski, sixty-one – a retired Polish teacher from Warsaw – sued the organisers of the 2003 World Sex Championships after they forgot to pixelate his face. The contest involved three young women having sex with as many men as they could over the course of several hours and Mr Szwerowski said he was left embarrassed when his young nephew saw him on a DVD of the event and told the rest of

IS IT IN YET?

his family. Demanding £2,500 in damages, Mr Szwerowski said, 'I was told that the faces of the participants would be blurred but this was not the case.'

In 1973 a family-planning organisation couldn't understand why the birth rate among Aboriginal women in South Australia was still rising, despite their best efforts at education: a memorable song that gave the women advice about contraception. It turned out the women thought that all they had to do to stop themselves becoming pregnant was to sing the song.

When Giovanni Vitale – a hot-blooded eighty-five-year-old Italian – discovered a very passionate and intimate love letter written to his wife, jealousy got the better of him. Seeing red, he stabbed his wife in the shoulder – only to later discover that the letter had actually been written by him, fifty years earlier.

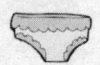

It's long been an urban myth that Coca-Cola makes an effective contraceptive douche... except it's not a myth. In a comprehensive research study, Deborah Anderson – a professor of obstetrics and gynaecology at Boston University's School of Medicine – put the claim to the test. To her and

MISCELLANEOUS

her colleague's surprise, it was true and their findings were published in *The New England Journal of Medicine* in 1985. For the record, Diet Coke worked best as a spermicide.

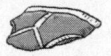

The Amazons – the nation of all-female warriors in Ancient Greece – were said to believe that lame men made the best lovers and would break the legs of any male prisoners they wanted to have sex with.

A Swedish woman unsuccessfully filed a paternity suit against Uri Geller, claiming that she'd fallen pregnant after watching one of his televised mind-bending exercises in 1974. She claimed he unravelled her copper IUD.

According to a report in *Australian Doctor* magazine, one in twenty men working on the production line in a contraceptive-pill factory developed breasts from absorbing oestrogen. Of the workers affected, one even began lactating, while others became impotent.

S&M

There's a certain degree of mystery and eroticism associated with the pain and passion of sadomasochism. However, you won't find it in the following incidents, where participants met inglorious ends as a result of dog leads, duct tape, gimp masks and cling film. It's hardly *Fifty Shades of Grey*...

In 2006 Lee Thompson – the leader of a bizarre sex-and-bondage cult known as the Kaotian sect – was banned from his local butcher's shop in Darlington, County Durham for taking his 'slave' in on a leash while he ordered bacon. Thompson, thirty-one, told the *Daily Record* about the sect, saying it 'works on the system that some women have a desire to serve.' Commenting on the sexual obligations of the slaves, he said, 'The girls do everything they are told when it comes to sex but it is all voluntary and safe.' Despite complaints from the public, since the slaves are volunteers, police were powerless to act.

IS IT IN YET?

A sixty-year-old grandmother from San Clemente, California, Betty Johnson Davies, who ran a 'sex dungeon', was arrested after a naked man was found choked to death with a dog leash around his neck in 1994. She told the court, 'We were just playing.' The man's death was ruled an accident and the Coroner's Office commented, 'Nobody forced him to be tied up and shackled in black leather.'

Australian Betty Wilson and her unnamed husband would play elaborate sex games that involved him being tied up for long periods of time. On one occasion, he was bound and gagged for ten hours before managing to escape. It all went wrong, however, in 2004, when Betty used rope and gaffer tape to tightly tie him to a bedpost and gag him. She went to take a shower and it was only afterwards that she discovered he'd suffocated. Appearing at a Brisbane court, where she was convicted of manslaughter, she commented, 'I told the fucking idiot he wouldn't get out of this one.'

You know that any story where someone has an unhealthy interest in mummification and bondage is not going to end well. Such it was with chef Alun Williams, who met Richard Bowler online and who visited his flat in Dover, Kent in August 2014 and asked to be wrapped head to toe in cling film and PVC sheeting. After being mummified this way, Williams accidentally died from a heart attack brought on by

S&M

drugs. After realising Williams wasn't moving or making any sounds, Bowler called 999 and told the operator, 'I thought he was just sleeping. I am sorry, I should have called before. He takes ketamine and that mongs him out.' Police who arrived at the flat discovered a series of sex toys, duct tape, a gas mask and ties. Bowler was sentenced to five years in prison for manslaughter.

A couple in Fort Lauderdale, Florida had handcuffed themselves to each other and then to the floor-to-ceiling bookcase in their bedroom. They were all set to take part in some bondage games when the husband dropped the key. The inquisitive family dog bounded over to see what was going on and, to the couple's horror, accidentally swallowed it. After a while, the couple managed to get themselves in a position where one of them could reach the phone. Police gained entry to their home to find them nude, handcuffed and extremely embarrassed.

In July 2011 forty-nine-year-old Sam Mozzola of Cleveland Ohio – owner of an exotic animal sanctuary – was found dead in his bedroom, handcuffed and chained to a waterbed, wearing a leather gimp mask zipped over his eyes and mouth and a two-piece metal sphere covering his head. The cause of death was suffocation, apparently after a sadomasochistic role-play went wrong; police found a sex toy lodged in his

IS IT IN YET?

throat. The Sheriff's department commented that the death 'was not suspicious.'

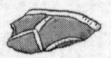

A fifty-five-year-old man from Burbank, California who was heavily into bondage, met a like-minded individual and arranged for a discipline session to take place at his apartment. The 'date' duly arrived and, according to his wishes, the man was stripped naked, spanked and then tightly tied to a 'discipline table' in his spare room. At this point, the date's accomplice arrived and, with their victim bound and helpless, the two of them proceeded to steal his stereo, his new TV and his sofa. They were never seen again.

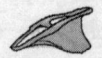

In September 2009 a couple from Basildon in Essex were involved in an intense bondage sex game when the woman became trapped in a pair of handcuffs. No matter how hard he tried, the man could not open them and, in his panic, he dialled 999 and asked the fire brigade if they could release his partner – however, to save their blushes, he begged them not to arrive with the siren blaring. After successfully freeing the woman, a fireman commented, 'They were very embarrassed, so we made a discreet entrance.'

S&M

In 2002 British Airways chiefs accused cabin crew of being 'fetishists' after hundreds of pairs of handcuffs went missing. In January of that year, the *Sunday Mirror* reported that a memo to all BA staff stated, 'Last year BA handcuffs were used to restrain 17 people but 255 handcuffs went missing! Now either that works out at 15 handcuffs per person restrained or we have a huge community of fetishists amongst crew.' The memo continued, 'Your exotic practices in the bedroom are your own business, but please stick to the Ann Summers furry handcuffs – replacing the ones from the restraint kit is costing BA a fortune.'

Commenting on the story, a BA spokeswoman said, 'Clearly our crew are so professional, they practise restraint procedures at home.'

Allan Pagan and his partner Natalie Fairhurst were walking with their two-year-old daughter near their home in Waterbeck, Dumfriesshire in October 2014, when they stumbled on a sight they'd rather forget: a man wearing leather bondage gear whipping a transvestite in a local country lane. After being surprised, both men jumped into a car and drove away at speed, almost knocking over Ms Fairhurst. Mr Pagan managed to get the vehicle's registration number and police were able to track down the driver: fifty-one-year-old David Wallace. The court heard how he was wearing a studded leather bondage collar as he thrashed the backside of an unknown man wearing a dress and blond wig. Wallace, of Workington, Cumbria admitted conducting

IS IT IN YET?

himself in a disorderly manner with the anonymous man, and to driving carelessly. He was fined £400. Police are still looking for the man in the wig.

STUCK!

From frankfurters to frozen fish, pencils to potatoes and even a Buzz Lightyear toy... There are only two things that limit the range of items that people insert into their bodies for sexual gratification: a) the capacity of the organ to accommodate them and b) the imagination of the person inserting the item...

Surgeons at Hospital Universitario in Londrina, southern Brazil had to perform a very delicate operation in order to remove a live South American lungfish from a man's intestine. The anonymous patient had decided to insert the fish into his anus to fulfil a bizarre sexual fantasy. However, the fish managed to wriggle its way into his guts before the man sought medical help. The lungfish can survive in environments with very little oxygen and was still alive when it was successfully removed. The operation was leaked onto social media and footage shows several medics in the operating theatre filming the operation, while raucous laughter can be heard in the background.

In August 2013 a seventy-year-old man was admitted to a Canberra hospital to have a fork removed from his urethra, after apparently inserting it for sexual gratification. According to news reports, the surgical team used forceps and 'copious lubrication' to remove the piece of cutlery while the patient was under general anaesthetic. The incident was reported in the *International Journal of Surgery Case Reports*, which commented, 'It is apparent that the human mind is uninhibited let alone creative.'

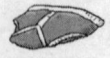

In February 2006 Zeljko Tupic from Belgrade, Serbia decided to try a novel technique to overcome his impotence. In order to maintain an erection, he stuck a narrow pencil down his urethra. The real problems started, however, when the pencil shifted and became lodged in his bladder, forcing him to cut the sex session short and call an ambulance.

Doctor Aleksandar Milosevic, from Belgrade's Zvezdara Hospital, who successfully removed the pencil, said, 'At first, the patient did not tell us what really happened but X-rays proved the truth. Tupic said he had no idea there were things like Viagra available but agreed that, in future, he will try pills before he takes any more chances with pencils.'

STUCK!

Officers from the Berowa Fire Rescue Service in New South Wales received an emergency call with a difference; they had to remove sixteen stainless-steel washers that a local resident had slid over his penis and couldn't remove. Professionals to the end, they didn't ask how (or why) the man had landed in this predicament and he was released by a combination of lubricant, brute force and delicately used cutting gear.

An unnamed girl from Munich visited her local clinic complaining of vaginal cramping. It was only when her legs were in the stirrups that her doctor found a frankfurter jammed in there.

A doctor at a Newport hospital reported a remarkably honest patient who presented himself with a carrot jammed firmly into his rectum. The seasoned doctor, who had, apparently, seen it all before, read the patient's notes and commented, 'I suppose you're going to tell me that you fell over while gardening naked or something along those lines?'

The patient shrugged and replied, 'No, nothing like that. I'm a sexual deviant.'

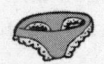

A woman who'd been arousing herself with a potato was horrified to find it had been pushed too far up her vagina for her to remove herself and she was too embarrassed to visit her doctor to see if he could retrieve it. After a few days, she plucked up the necessary courage and the potato was successfully removed but not before it had grown a stalk of about six inches; the warm, dark and moist conditions were perfect for germination.

An American man with severe abdominal pains was admitted for surgery and, while being prepped, surgeons noticed the tip on an unidentified blue object poking out from his penis that looked like the end of a piece of string. Examination of the patient's bladder revealed that it was completely filled with about six feet of knotted nylon jump rope. The man had decided to remove the handles and slowly pass the knotted rope bit by bit into his urethra, pulling it slowly out for a sexual thrill. The rope however, had knotted about itself in his bladder, making removal impossible without surgery.

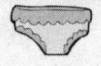

In August 2008 police and medical personnel were called to Lan Tian Park in Hong Kong. Forty-one-year-old local man Le Xing had got into difficulty after he put his penis through a hole in the bench and got stuck once he became aroused. He had to be taken to hospital with the 2.5-metre bench still attached to him and it took doctors four hours to cut him free. Staff at the hospital later said that, if he had been stuck for just an hour longer, they might have been

STUCK!

forced to amputate his penis. When questioned as to how he'd ended up in the predicament, Mr Xing decided that honesty was the best policy and simply told police that he thought it would be fun to have sex with a park bench. He was described as a 'lonely and disturbed man.'

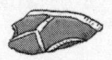

Forget cucumbers, carrots and bananas, even vibrators and candles; they're positively prosaic compared to some of the more exotic objects that have been officially reported by medical authorities as being surgically removed from embarrassed patients. Here follows a list of examples.
- French bread
- Cigarette lighter
- Umbrella handle
- Frozen pig's tail
- Soldering iron
- Miniature ice pick
- Bottle of Coke
- Tin of condensed milk
- Whisky bottle
- Artillery shell
- Half-full tobacco pouch
- Sand-filled bicycle inner tube
- Teacup
- Jar of peanut butter (crunchy variety)
- Light bulb
- Pair of spectacles
- Oil can

IS IT IN YET?

- Screwdriver
- Seventy-two fine jewellers' saws (all from the same patient)
- Torch
- Pint glass
- Mobile phone
- Pistol
- Live eel
- Whisk
- Cassette tape
- Salad tongs (which became stuck trying to remove a
- vibrator)
- Sunglasses
- Barbie doll
- Can of shaving cream
- Buzz Lightyear toy
- Copy of the *Church Times*

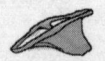

A middle-aged man went to his local ER complaining of severe abdominal pain and rectal bleeding. It didn't take long for the doctor on call to realise the reason: the patient had a coat hanger protruding from his rectum. After recovering from an emergency bowel resection, the man explained what had happened. Earlier that night, when his wife was at work, he wanted to 'pleasure himself' and impulsively pushed an uncooked egg into his anus. When it became lost 'up there', he panicked and tried to fish it out with the coat hanger. When this became snagged he decided the best thing would be to try and shake it out, using the vibrations from his

STUCK!

motorbike. However, riding his motorbike all the way to the ER just pushed it further in.

When fifty-year-old Nigel Willis of Forest Hill in London got a vibrating butt plug lodged in his bottom in December 2013, he was too embarrassed to seek medical help. It was only after he confessed to a friend that the sex aid had been stuck there and buzzing away for five days that he was persuaded to go to hospital. Unfortunately, by then it was too late. He was rushed in on New Year's Eve and admitted to intensive care with septic shock and underwent emergency surgery to remove what the hospital called a 'foreign body' from his anus. He died on 7 February 2014. A post-mortem examination determined the cause of death to be multi-organ failure, sepsis and a perforated bowel.

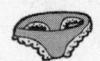

Paramedics rushed to the home of a San Francisco man who admitted over the phone that he'd done something 'really stupid'. He wasn't joking – the medics found a fish stuck in his rectum. It turned out that the man had thrust the frozen fish, head first, up his bottom but, after the first few thrusts, it had begun to thaw and the dorsal fin had extended, jamming the fish in place.

IS IT IN YET?

An article in an American medical journal in 1990 recounts the story of a twenty-nine-year-old woman who visited a clinic complaining of missing her period. On examination, the doctor discovered 'a cylindrical mass of pale grey tissue' lodged in the woman's vagina. After further questioning, the patient admitted that this was a preserved deer tongue that she used for masturbation. She confessed that her husband was a hunter and that, after he'd gutted the deer in their garage, she'd seen the tongue, admired its length and had sneaked off to use it as a masturbatory aid – though she didn't remember leaving it up there.

A man from Inverness was so sexually frustrated that he decided to have sex with a glass milk bottle. It was, apparently, quite pleasurable at first – and then his penis got stuck in the neck. The man tried using butter as a lubricant to release himself, then hit upon the not-so-bright idea of pouring boiling water over the bottle to make it expand and release him. Needless to say, the boiling water heated the bottle so it was unbearable and the man, in agony, smashed it. He was admitted to hospital with a bleeding, scalded penis, complete with the bottleneck still in place – oh, yes, and lots of glass splinters.

In February 2001 a Taiwanese man redefined the phrase 'phone sex'. The man called his girlfriend on his Nokia

STUCK!

8850 mobile phone... nothing unusual in that, you might think, except that she'd inserted the phone up her bottom so that she'd be stimulated by the vibrating ring-tone. The whole episode ended in embarrassment, however, when the phone slipped too far up inside the woman and couldn't be retrieved. After experiencing severe abdominal pains, the woman was forced to visit the Taipei Medical University Hospital, where the phone was eventually removed. A Nokia spokesman commented, 'We can't control how the users use their phones. It's just a personal issue.'

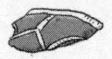

If you're in a gym and you see a barbell weight lying on the floor, do you automatically think, 'I wonder if my dick will fit in that hole?' Most people wouldn't but an anonymous gym member from Wichita, Kansas decided to put it to the test. It did fit but the excitement of finding out caused the man to have an erection, resulting in the weight becoming firmly stuck. The man had to be taken to hospital with the weight, where a urologist had to drain blood from his penis to remove the item.

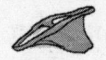

A thirty-eight-year-old woman presented herself at the Aberdeen Royal Infirmary showing signs of infection and severe emaciation. An examination by staff revealed that she had a five-inch vibrator pressing on her bladder, which was responsible for urine painfully collecting in her kidneys.

IS IT IN YET?

The vibrator was surgically removed but what was more surprising than the sex toy becoming stuck was how long it had actually been there. The woman said she recalled inserting the toy ten years before but could not remember if she had removed it or not.

Replacing his wife's perfume was the least of the problems of a thirty-nine-year-old Wisconsin lawyer. His biggest issue was explaining how her bottle of body spray had become stuck up his anus in the first place. The 17 x 3 cm object was finally removed in hospital after a spinal anaesthetic was given to the man and, according to the doctor's report, 'The patient was released on the second postoperative day. He refused psychological counselling.' The name of the perfume? Impulse.

Watching a porn film where a live eel is inserted into someone's rectum is one thing – copying the act is quite another matter. A thirty-nine-year-old man did just that to himself but lost his grip and the eel slithered straight up into his bowels. Panicking, the man presented himself at his nearest A&E, bursting through the door and shouting the not-very-often heard phrase, 'Help me. An eel is moving through my body.' After establishing the fact that the man wasn't hallucinating or mad, it took the duty surgeon an hour to successfully coax the creature out with a suction machine.

STUCK!

It's not often that firefighters become surgeons but it happened in October 2008 in the city of Newburgh, New York. They were called to St Luke's Cornwall Hospital and asked to bring equipment to remove a ring. When they arrived, they discovered that their ring cutter – used to remove wedding bands from swollen fingers – wouldn't be enough. They also discovered that the seventy-three-year-old male patient that they had been called to attend to didn't have a ring stuck on his finger – he had a steel pipe stuck on his penis that was made of quarter-inch-thick steel. He'd been using it as an artificial vagina. The man's penis was swollen and was turning purple so a rapid removal was vital. The only tool to do the job was a pneumatic saw, usually used by emergency responders at the scene of car crashes. After what seemed like an eternity (it took five bottles of compressed air), the saw clipped through the final piece of pipe and the victim was freed. He is reported to have pleaded with the nervous firefighter carrying out the operation, 'Just don't cut it off.'

An elderly man was admitted to hospital with a cock ring (for those who don't know, it's used to slow the flow of blood and therefore maintain an erection) firmly stuck behind his scrotum, causing the scrotum and penis to swell to four times their usual size. The consultant urologist who examined him was surprised to hear that the man had been like this for three days. When asked why he hadn't gone to hospital earlier, the patient said he didn't think there was any real emergency; he could still urinate and his wife was happy!

IS IT IN YET?

An unnamed twenty-two-year-old man from Brighton arrived at the busy A&E department of the Royal Sussex County Hospital suffering from severe pelvic pain. The reason became immediately apparent after an X-ray: several small balls lodged in his bladder. How they got there was quite simple really. The man had been getting himself aroused by sliding a small necklace in and out of his penis. All was fine until the thread snapped and the beads disappeared. A delicate operation was needed to remove each bead separately by tweezers.

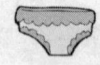

NOT TONIGHT, DARLING...

The following are stories of virginity, celibacy or just not being in the mood. Like the married couple that waited fourteen years to have sex and then died of shock from the experience. And the man who set fire to his own house just so he wouldn't have to sleep with his wife...

A couple from Berlin – Hans and Heidi Berger – filed for divorce, citing lack of sex for the breakdown in their marriage. She was 100 and he was 101.

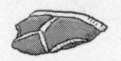

In September 2003 Svetin Gulisija – a twenty-six-year-old man from Seget, Croatia – was too tired to have sex, so he decided to distract his wife. Unfortunately, the method he chose was starting a fire in woods behind their house. Fanned by winds, the fire soon got out of control and their house was badly burned. Gulisija was subsequently sentenced to two years in prison for criminal damage.

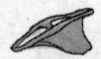

When Maithrey Mohan of Orpington, Kent got married at the age of twenty-seven, she'd never been told the facts of life. She wasn't worried though, as she was confident that her thirty-three-year-old groom would be more experienced. He wasn't. Totally confused on their wedding night, they had to resort to calling Maithrey's parents to find out what they should be doing. After a brief lecture and copious note taking, they successfully consummated the marriage.

Tina and Paul Haswell were given some sage advice from Barking and Dagenham Council when they complained about damp in their flat. Their housing manager told them to stop having sex because their heavy breathing was responsible for increased condensation in the apartment.

Howard Hughes gave up sex completely in his mid-fifties because of his paranoid fear of germs.

NOT TONIGHT, DARLING...

A policy of sex-education lessons in Texas schools that promoted abstinence didn't prove that successful. A study showed that 23 per cent of ninth-grade girls (fourteen to fifteen years old) had already had sex by the time they received the abstinence lessons. After the lessons, this percentage actually rose.

When Cesare Borgia – son of Pope Alexander VI – married Charlotte D'Albret in 1499, his wedding night was a disaster. A court practical joker substituted his normal medication for strong laxatives.

After Napoleon Bonaparte divorced Josephine, he married Princess Marie Louise of Austria. On their wedding night, not only did he discover she was a virgin but that she had never actually seen a male sex organ before. Her parents were so protective of her that they even kept male animals out of her sight.

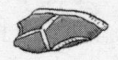

Ten famous people suspected of dying a virgin:
- Elizabeth I
- Sir Isaac Newton
- Mother Teresa
- J. Edgar Hoover

IS IT IN YET?

- George Bernard Shaw
- Joan of Arc
- Adolf Hitler
- Nikola Tesla
- Lewis Carroll
- Hans Christian Andersen

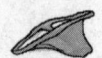

Elvira Babsezian of Stuttgart was so frustrated with her sexually inactive husband that she decided to look further afield for sexual gratification. She placed an anonymous note in her local paper saying 'Sex kitten seeks sharp cat.' She was stunned to see that among the replies was one from her husband, who'd included a nude photo of himself wearing cat ears. Elvira commented, 'It was the first time I have seen him naked in fourteen years of marriage.'

An anonymous twenty-eight-year-old man divorced his wife on the grounds that he found it impossible to have sex with her, due to the five little words she insisted on uttering when he was about to climax. This started two months after they got married and, according to the man, 'I begged her never to use the phrase again. I pleaded with her!' The five little words were, 'Give it all to mummy.'

NOT TONIGHT, DARLING...

In July 2001 an anonymous eighteen-year-old Romanian woman resented the fact that her husband, Mircea Stoleru, returned home one night and fell asleep without having sex with her. To show her displeasure, she took a hot iron and burned him with it. Mircea later accepted that he was to blame for his wife's actions, saying, 'This should serve me right. I knew what I would get when I married such a young and beautiful wife.'

The wife of a local government official in Cologne claimed she could only have sex with her husband when she heard the sound of church bells – and they had to be real bells; a recording didn't work for her. This meant they could only make love on Sunday mornings or when there were weddings. A court granted him a divorce.

Erwin Gehlen's wife would only let her husband have sex if he successfully answered a series of riddles. These became harder as the years passed and he told a divorce court in Stockholm, 'It finally reached the stage when I was lucky to solve three a year.'

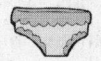

IS IT IN YET?

Noted British stage and film actor Sir Cedric Hardwicke dealt with his impotence in good humour, introducing himself as 'Sir Seldom Hardprick'.

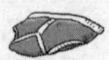

Sex researchers estimate that around 7 per cent of married couples have never had sex.

A young Japanese couple, Sachi and Tomio Hidaki, were married in 1978 but both were so inexperienced and shy that it took fourteen years before they decided to consummate their marriage. Unfortunately, the excitement of having sex for the first time proved too great and they both died from shock.

It's widely reported that, on his wedding night in 1848, John Ruskin – the renowned Victorian author and art critic – found the sight of his wife Effie's pubic hair so shocking that he vowed never to sleep with her again. Due to non-consummation, the marriage was annulled six years later. Ruskin's biographer, Mary Lutyens, suggests that Ruskin could have been traumatised because he'd only known the female form through Greek statues and nude paintings, which always omitted the pubic hair.

NOT TONIGHT, DARLING...

In the Middle Ages, it was believed that venereal disease could be cured by having sex with a virgin.

A Croatian man really, really didn't want have sex with his wife – so much so, in fact, that, to get out of his marital duties, he set fire to his own house. After admitting his involvement in the fire – and the reason – he received a two-year prison sentence and a bill for the equivalent of £15,000.

Confirmed celibate Mahatma Gandhi used to regularly sleep with young naked women to prove to himself that he could not be tempted.

Marie Antoinette and King Louis XVI took seven years to consummate their marriage, his presumed impotence making them the laughing stock of the royal court.

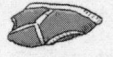

According to a report in the *Journal of Sexual Medicine*, it took a young couple from Huntington called Rosemary and Alan two years before they consummated their marriage. The problem was a lack of privacy. At first, they lived with Rosemary's parents and they were convinced that their

IS IT IN YET?

lovemaking would be overheard. After that, they inherited and moved into her grandparents' house but on the condition they kept on the old lodger that lived there. They were convinced he, too, would overhear them. Frustrated, they had counselling to overcome their anxiety but, at the crucial moment when they were about to have sex, they heard their lodger scream and die from a heart attack.

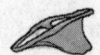

Staunch anti-masturbation campaigner and cereal pioneer John Harvey Kellogg spent his wedding night with his bride Ella Eaton in 1879 writing his book *Plain Facts For Old and Young*: his detailed treatise on the evils of sexual intercourse. Unsurprisingly, the marriage was never consummated.

Although short and ugly, tyrant Attila the Hun had a procession of wives… though his wedding night to bride number twelve was very short-lived. During energetic and drunken lovemaking, she accidentally hit him in the face, breaking his nose. He died from a subsequent haemorrhage.

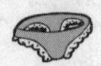

In June 1831 Moses Alexander, aged 93, married Frances Tompkins, 105. They were found dead in their bed the next day.

SEX LAWS

It's difficult to know what's more bizarre: the fact that these American state and local laws were actually proposed and passed in the first place, or that many of them still stand. That said, if you own more than six dildos in Mississippi, you're unlikely to be arrested…

- It's illegal for a man and a woman to have sex in an ambulance (Tremont, Utah).
- You're not permitted to buy a sex toy on Valentine's Day (Alabama).
- A woman cannot strip off in front of a picture of a man (Ohio).
- You may not have more than two dildos in a house (Arizona).
- It is illegal for a man to kiss his wife on Sunday (Hartford, Connecticut).

IS IT IN YET?

- Women may walk in public topless, provided they have their nipples covered (New Mexico).
- You may not kiss your wife's breasts (Florida).
- It's illegal to own more than six dildos (Mississippi).
- All sex toys are banned (Georgia).
- Anyone arrested for soliciting a hooker must have their name and picture shown on television (Oklahoma).
- It's illegal to have sexual relations with a porcupine (Florida).
- A woman cannot be on top during sexual activities (Massachusetts).
- Couples are banned from making love in an automobile unless the act takes place while the vehicle is parked on the couple's own property (Michigan).
- Persons with gonorrhoea may not marry (Nebraska).
- Nudity is allowed, provided that male genitals are covered (New Mexico).
- It's against the law to kiss a woman that is sleeping (Colorado).
- Women must have their bodies covered by at least sixteen yards of cloth at all times (Charlotte, North Carolina).
- It is illegal for the owner of a bar to allow anyone inside to pretend to have sex with a buffalo (Oklahoma).
- You need a doctor's note before you can purchase a sex toy (Georgia).
- It's illegal to possess realistic dildos (Dallas, Texas).
- It is illegal to tickle women (Virginia).
- A man may face sixty days in jail for patting a woman's derriere (Norfolk, Virginia).
- It is legal for a male to have sex with an animal, as long as it does not exceed 40 lbs (West Virginia).

SEX LAWS

- All couples staying overnight in a hotel must have a room with double beds that are at least two feet apart (North Carolina).
- It is illegal to kiss on a train (Wisconsin).
- It's illegal to dress as a penis if conducting official state business (Nevada).
- You cannot have sex inside a premise's walk-in meat freezer (Newcastle, Wyoming).
- A man may not shoot a firearm while his female partner is having an orgasm (Connorsville, Wisconsin).
- It's illegal to have sex with a truck driver at a toll booth (Harrisburg, Pennyslvania).
- You're forbidden from talking dirty in your wife's ear (Willowdale, Oregon).
- You're not allowed to masturbate while watching two people have sex in a car (Clinton, Oklahoma).

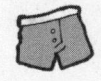

FOOD FUN AND GAMES

The use of food in lovemaking can be incredibly sensual – but not when the act involves a royal employee doing something unnatural with a jar of Bovril, a man exposing himself with Swiss cheese wrapped around his penis, or someone making love to a burning hot lasagne (and instantly regretting it)...

Steven Brown of California would enhance his orgasm by getting his girlfriend to hit him in the face with a pie at the point of ejaculation. After he was dumped he would gatecrash local social functions and ask female guests to do the same thing to him. Oh, yes... he describes himself as a piesexual.

Taking inspiration from an online video of a man having sex with a homemade lasagne, forty-seven-year-old Vince Shaw

IS IT IN YET?

of Winsford, Cheshire bought a 95p Tesco Value Lasagne, popped it in the microwave for ten minutes and then inserted his penis into microwaved meal. As a result, he spent two days in Leighton hospital recovering from severe genital scalds. Mr Shaw told the *Sunday Sport* newspaper, 'After two weeks, I was allowed to take the bandages off. Good God – my bell end looks like cheese on toast!' At the time of writing, Mr Shaw was considering legal action against the supermarket chain, commenting, 'When I paid for it, the checkout girl did not say, "Do not have sex with this product when it is piping hot."'

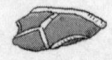

Dubbed the 'Swiss Cheese Pervert', forty-two-year-old Christopher Pagano from Pennsylvania pleaded guilty in June 2014 to driving around town, exposing himself and then offering women money to put cheese on his penis. The court heard how he wrote to a woman he met online: 'I love the way Swiss cheese feels against my penis, either as slices of Swiss cheese being wrapped around my penis or a chunk of Swiss cheese being rubbed against my penis.' During the hearing, Pagano admitted stalking, indecent exposure, harassment and lewdness charges against four women. The married father was sentenced to eight years' probation and has to report for sex-offender counselling. He was also banned from driving. When pressed on his preferences, Pagano told the court, 'I don't like cheese, except for mozzarella, and that's the one cheese I have never used on myself.' He also cleared up one question: 'No, I do not eat the cheese after I am done using it for pleasure; it is discarded.'

FOOD FUN AND GAMES

A twenty-one-year-old Ohio woman who was woken by the sounds of burglars leaving her home was shocked to discover that they had covered her buttocks with whipped cream and sugar.

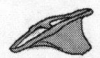

Just before the start of the fire that ripped through Windsor Castle in November 1992, a caretaker was arrested for performing an undisclosed sex act with a jar of Bovril in the Queen's private chapel – where the fire began.

Thirty-two-year-old David Joseph Zaba of Denver and his wife Angela had used food to spice up their sex life for about six years. In one session, in March 1995, instead of the honey and chocolate syrup she'd been expecting to have poured over her, Mr Zaba instead covered his wife with varnish, which later made her hair fall out. In June he pleaded guilty to a charge of assault. The court heard how he'd used varnish before but that, this time, Angela had had enough so she called the police.

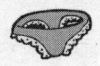

In 1981 an intruder entered a woman's apartment in Virginia Beach, Virginia and assaulted her in a very peculiar and specific way: he rubbed chocolate and vanilla cake icing all over her face and clothes. Before he escaped, he told his shocked victim that she should have expected this would happen when she left her doors unlocked.

A British man used to pleasure himself by having sex with a melon. All was good until he decided to make it feel more authentically like a vagina. The answer, he thought, was to warm it in a microwave. The result was second-degree burns to his penis. When later questioned, the anonymous victim commented, 'I used oven gloves to protect my hands but I didn't think about my bobby.'

A similar fate befell seventeen-year-old Dwight Emburger, who was rushed to hospital in Boise, Idaho in March 2000 with a scalded penis after trying to recreate 'that scene' from one of the *American Pie* films. He'd been too impatient to wait for the boiling pie filling to cool down first.

An anonymous man was arrested by store detectives at his local supermarket. He wasn't shoplifting though. He would get sexually aroused by poking and squeezing the bread on display.

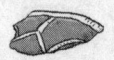

A Dutchman was arrested for stealing from a sex shop in Utrecht. Surprisingly, he wasn't interested in any of the expensive merchandise on display. On multiple occasions, he'd been caught shoplifting miniature chocolate penises.

FOR THE THRILL OF IT

For some people, the actual satisfaction derived from a sexual act is outweighed by the thrill of doing something bizarre, dangerous or illegal – or all three. That's why you'll find a couple who had sex on train tracks, a man who exposed himself in a bear enclosure and the woman who could only achieve orgasm by shoplifting...

In September 2013 a Ukrainian couple decided to have a spontaneous fling on a railway track early one Saturday morning. Caught up in the moment, they failed to hear an approaching train and the driver couldn't stop in time. The incident resulted in the woman being killed and her boyfriend losing his legs. He later told police in Zaporozhye that they had 'failed to overcome their natural passion when walking home ... and wanted to experience an extreme sensation near the railroad tracks.'

IS IT IN YET?

Retired German electrician Manfred Lubitz was found dead in his Malaga apartment wearing a handmade contraption he called the 'Orgasmatron'. This device featured a vibrating mat, massage pads and electrodes attached to his penis. Police believe he was electrocuted after a sudden power surge.

A young Mexican couple, Jose and Ana-Maria, decided to add a frisson of excitement to their love life by having sex in the car Jose drove for the Perez Diaz funeral home in Campeche. They drove to a nearby warehouse and went ahead with their sex session, leaving the car's engine running so the air conditioning would cool them off. They forgot about the dangers of carbon monoxide poisoning and it wasn't long before they died from suffocation – appropriately enough, in the back of a hearse.

A twenty-three-year-old woman named only as 'Debbi Anne' was arrested in British Colombia, Canada in 1994 after a car chase that reached speeds of up to 120 mph. She told the arresting officers that she suffered from what she called a 'sexual speed fetish' and had an overwhelming urge to play with herself while driving recklessly fast, stating, 'I can only come when I smell the aroma of hot tyres.' She was ordered to get immediate psychiatric help or face jail.

FOR THE THRILL OF IT

In June 1993 a married couple pleaded 'no contest' to a charge of public indecency after engaging in sex in a booth in a family restaurant in New Philadelphia, Ohio. At their hearing, the judge said the couple should grow up and act their age. The couple were sixty and seventy years old.

When twenty-nine-year-old Kirsten Taylor of Craley, Pennsylvania died from electrocution, her husband, Toby, initially told the police she'd been shocked by her hairdryer. Medical examination proved that this was not the case, at which point he admitted she'd been killed by a malfunctioning electric nipple clamp. It transpired that the couple had been engaging in what he called 'electric shock sex' for about two years and, on the night she died, he was stimulating her by repeatedly turning the current on and off. Unfortunately, something went wrong and one of the shocks killed her.

In October 2007 forty-seven-year-old Christopher Harris of Newport in Wales was found dead in the bedroom of his home, still wearing a Soviet Union military-issue gas mask. An inquest at Newport Coroner's Court heard that Mr Harris's particular fetish was to take pain; a friend of his said he sometimes used face masks and breath deprivation in order to get a kick. When Mr Harris's body was found, the gas mask was connected by a tube to a bottle of chloroform. A verdict of misadventure was recorded.

IS IT IN YET?

Early one morning in October 2008 police in Saginaw County, Michigan were called to investigate reports of someone acting suspiciously at a car wash in Swan Creek Township. There they found twenty-nine-year-old Jason L. Savage 'receiving sexual favours from a vacuum.' He pleaded 'no contest' to indecent exposure and was sentenced to ninety days in jail. The officer who caught Mr Savage commented, 'I've seen some strange things but this is the weirdest one…'

Justin Call and Tina Gianakon of Kansas decided to steal a bottle of sexual lubricant from their local Walmart. However, rather than stop there, they decided to test it by having full intercourse in the aisle, right in front of the store's many customers. Police were called to arrest the couple and an officer later commented that the most surprising part of the story was that the couple were both completely sober.

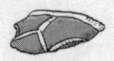

In June 1999 police were on patrol in Newtown, Powys when they spotted a group of teenagers excitedly watching some activity across the other side of a river. Further observation showed this to be Jennifer Visser, twenty-one, and her boyfriend Craig Watkins, eighteen, having sex on a picnic table in a local beauty spot. The couple were arrested and charged with causing alarm and distress but pleaded guilty by letter, as they were too embarrassed to appear at Newtown Magistrates Court. Both were fined £120, with £35 costs.

FOR THE THRILL OF IT

After the hearing, an officer commented, 'Even though they were enjoying a private moment, it was in a very public place and could clearly have caused great offence.'

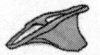

A picnic table had a similar allure for fifty-five-year-old Larry Wayne Williamson, who was arrested in October 2008 on charges of public indecency and public nudity in the town of Evansville, Indiana. Witnesses observed Mr Williamson sitting at a picnic table in Scott Township Park, completely naked and committing a sex act. Police searched his car, which was parked nearby, and discovered a selection of sex toys, binoculars, male enhancement pills, energy pills, marijuana, a 'variety of other suspicious and unusual items' — and a small dog that desperately wanted to go for walk.

It probably seemed like a good idea at the time but Andrew Farlow now rues that fateful day in 2001 when he suggested involving the pet dog in his sex games. Andrew and his wife were larking around in the bedroom when he suggested that he spread peanut butter on his genitals and get his pooch to lick it off. The overexcited (and hungry) dog nipped Andrew's penis in the process, causing Rosemary to throw a bottle of perfume at it. This enraged the dog even more and it bit her husband again — even more fiercely this time. That signalled the end of their sexual experimentation.

IS IT IN YET?

If you're going to join the mile-high club, it makes sense to do it discreetly; not by stripping to your bra and knickers and performing a sex act in Club Class in front of astonished fellow passengers. This is what happened in October 1999 when thirty-six-year-old Mandy Holt met forty-year-old David Machin on board an American Airlines flight from Dallas to Manchester. Both were married to other partners and they'd never met before the flight but, 30,000 feet above the Atlantic, they engaged in their 'sex romp'. Airline staff alerted police and the pair were arrested on landing and taken to police cells. The story subsequently appeared in several national newspapers, leading Mrs Holt's solicitor to comment, 'This incident has caused a great deal of distress, both to this lady, her family and friends. I would hope – and she would hope – that you can give some consideration for that.' When confronted by reporters at his home, Mr Machin said, 'I can't say anything at all. I am in trouble already over this.'

As a result of the incident and the attendant publicity, the pair lost their jobs. At their hearing, both admitted to being drunk on board an aircraft and were subsequently fined but were spared a jail sentence. One of Mrs Holt's neighbours told the press, 'She never wore anything tarty or anything to make you think she's that kind of girl.'

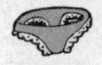

A security guard at a factory that manufactured piñatas was captured on CCTV leaving his post and having sex with a dog-shaped piñata. He later claimed that the papier-mâché pooch had been put there as a form of entrapment, claiming, 'I think they purposely put the dog in there to lure me in.'

An Australian man accidentally drowned his twenty-five-year-old companion after she gave him a blow job underwater. He held her underwater too long and only released her when he climaxed. He later told authorities that he had confused her death throes with signs of passion.

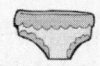

In what's become an apocryphal tale, two men were admitted to Salt Lake City Hospital with severe burns after some kinky animal fun got out of hand. It started when one of the men decided he wanted to experience what it would be like to have a gerbil inserted in his anus. A cardboard tube was duly inserted between his buttocks and the gerbil slipped in and was encouraged to go deep. Curious, the friend peered down the tube and lit a match so he could see the rodent's progress. Unfortunately, this ignited a pocket of intestinal gas, with the effect that the gerbil was forcibly expelled and the two men suffered severe burns: one to his lower intestinal tract and the other to his face... also sustaining a broken nose from the impact of the ejected gerbil.

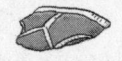

IS IT IN YET?

Elizabeth Hooper and Jeff Healey crept into Windsor Great Park for a sex romp in August 1994 and decided what they needed to do to get into the mood was to strip naked and climb a large oak tree. In the process, Elizabeth slipped and fell to the ground. Jeff shimmied down, hastily dressed and ran off. She was found by a Crown Estates ranger, naked and writhing in agony with a broken leg, and was taken to a hospital in Slough.

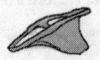

Julie Amiri of Staines, Middlesex had a novel defence when she was arrested for shoplifting from two department stores in July 1993. The thirty-five-year-old British divorcee told the court that stealing and being chased and arrested by police officers was the only way she could reach orgasm. In support of her claim, her psychologist told the court that 'uniforms, police interviews, flashing blue lights and sirens all turned her on,' while Amiri herself admitted, 'I had my first orgasm in the back of a police car, aged twenty-eight. After that, I was around the shops every day.'

The judge didn't believe her defence and she was fined £200.

In June 2008 an Italian couple were cautioned for indulging in an obscene public act and for disturbing a religious ceremony. Their crime? Having oral sex in the confessional box at Cesena Cathedral. In their defence, they claimed they were atheists and that 'having sex in church is just like having it in any other place.'

Mr Kynham Dudley certainly liked a little bit of excitement in his life, leaping over a wall and into the bear enclosure at London Zoo, where he exposed himself to the dangerous animals. Zookeepers rescued and detained him until the police arrived. On being arrested, Mr Dudley shouted in defiance, 'No one will stop me flashing!' The zoo's bear keeper, Mr Bob Tuffy, commented, 'When Rusty and Jumble were flashed, they just walked away. They were disgusted.'

When the Selfridges department store in Birmingham opened for business one day in 2003, the last thing staff in the bedding department expected to witness was a four-in-a-bed sex romp – particularly when three of the bed's occupants were store mannequins. Aydin Demir had broken into the store during the night, removed the dummies from the shop floor and taken them to bed with him. He was subsequently charged with burglary and criminal damage.

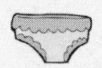

IS IT IN YET?

Two lovers in the village of Brnicko in the Czech Republic wanted the thrill of having sex in the open air and thought they'd found the perfect location: the darkened corner of a field. They forgot it was harvest time and were run over by the farmer's tractor.

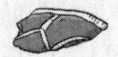

SEX FOR SALE

The 'Oldest Profession' is also the weirdest. If you doubt this, read on about the man who paid a prostitute to allow him to pelt her with kippers, the man who haggled so much with a hooker that he had a heart attack and the bus driver who went kerb crawling – in his double-decker bus...

In 1990 Franco Stella – a thirty-five-year-old Italian lorry driver – was given the address of an exclusive brothel in the town of Teramo by a close friend. The friend also recommended one particular hooker there. This turned out to be Franco's wife, Anna, who had been secretly working there at night.

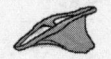

IS IT IN YET?

In June 2008 a prostitute in Reno, Nevada chose the wrong person to proposition: a veteran homicide detective. Although he was sitting in an unmarked police car, there was a flashing light on the dashboard and a blaring police radio. After he pointed out that he was a detective, the prostitute is said to have commented, 'Oh. I didn't think police officers wore glasses.'

A forty-one-year-old high-school teacher admitted paying students to swear at him, spit in his face, urinate and defecate on him. Investigators who searched his apartment and computer said he contacted his first victims via MySpace and that it didn't take long for word to spread that the teens could get paid to spit in a man's face.

A drunken thirty-three-year-old Thai man was badly bitten by a dog on his face, chest and arms after he'd tried to have sex with it. Police were called when residents saw the man staggering down the street, bleeding. The man told police that he turned to the dog after he realised he didn't have enough money to visit a prostitute.

One of the first recorded cases of autoerotic asphyxiation was that of the famous Czech composer and virtuoso double-

SEX FOR SALE

bassist Frantisek Kotzwara, who died in London in 1791. He tied his neck with a ligature to a doorknob and suffocated while having sex with a prostitute. The girl in question, Susannah Hill, was acquitted of his death and told the Old Bailey that, before they had sex, she'd refused the troubled musician's request to cut off his testicles.

In January 2012 a woman was arrested in Burbank, Los Angeles on suspicion of prostitution, after she accosted men in the drive-thru lane at a McDonald's, offering to perform oral sex in exchange for Chicken McNuggets.

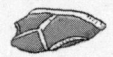

Not so much sex for sale as grades for groping, Arthur Miller – a University of Iowa professor – offered female students better grades if they let him see them topless, or if he could lick or fondle their breasts. The complaints began in May 2008. One student told police that, during a meeting with Miller, he said she wasn't doing well. He then, allegedly, told her she would 'have to do something for him.' She said Miller then grabbed and sucked on her breast. She later received an email from Miller congratulating her on her A+ grade and offering her more assistance with getting into law school. The professor was later found dead in Hickory Park in August, having shot himself with a rifle he'd bought two months earlier.

IS IT IN YET?

When bus driver Cristoval Guiarro decided to go kerb crawling, he chose a very conspicuous type of vehicle: his red double-decker bus. Undercover police stopped his number 57 bus and arrested him after watching him stop and pick up a prostitute along his route in Streatham, South London in 2003.

Forty-three-year-old Kelly Cooper of Maricopa County, Arizona was so desperate for petrol that she offered a male attendant at a gas station sex in exchange. During negotiations, the deal went wrong and Cooper ended up assaulting the attendant with a pair of scissors. After her arrest, Cooper described her scheme as 'a sex-for-gas contract gone bad.'

After visiting a German brothel, a man hired the services of a twenty-four-year-old prostitute called 'Priya'. She teased him by removing her clothes really slowly and seductively and it wasn't long before the client was 'sweaty with excitement', waiting for his reward after a long day at work. It was only when Priya was completely naked that the client realised she was actually a transsexual – in effect, a man who feels he's a woman trapped in a man's body.

At this revelation, the client became dizzy and collapsed. The coroner's report stated that he died of a heart attack from the shock exacerbated by excessive use of Viagra.

SEX FOR SALE

An unidentified elderly Croatian man was negotiating the price of a blow job with a thirty-year-old prostitute. The haggling went on for ages, with the man getting more and more animated. Eventually, he wore the prostitute down to the equivalent of £5 but he was so excited by his bargaining and this rock-bottom price that, as he dropped his trousers, he died from a heart attack.

One Japanese prostitute working from a boat offered a special service to her clients. She would lean over the side and dunk her head in the water. Her clients, meanwhile, would enter her from behind and enjoy the rectal spasms as she almost drowned. One day, however, she did.

Prostitutes have reported the following odd requests made of them by clients in order to get sexual thrills: throw a pie in their face, pelt them with orange peel and dress up as Mr Blobby.

After jailing members of a prostitution ring in Xiangzhou, China, a spokesman from the vice squad reported that the women were all over seventy, the oldest being ninety-three. Apart from prostitution being illegal, the women were also charged with contravening the terms of their pension by continuing to work.

IS IT IN YET?

Services offered included oral sex, with clients paying a third more if they wanted women to remove their false teeth.

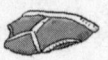

Until the early 1980s, a one-legged prostitute was operating in the San Francisco area who claimed to have 'more business than [she] could handle.'

According to Lord Kennet's classic 1964 book *Eros Denied*, some of the weirder requests by clients to prostitutes included someone who made her stand naked while he threw kippers wrapped in cellophane at her and someone who made the girl sit naked with her legs apart on the other side of the room while he threw cream buns at her. The book also records a man who liked being chained down and having hot wax poured over his penis. He was an MP.

A Bulgarian woman would scam men by beckoning to them from a rowboat moored just off the shore of a deserted lake. As men approached, they'd notice the lower part of her bikini tied to one of the oars – a definite signal of what she wanted. The men would get in the boat and row to the middle of the lake and have sex with the woman. As soon as they'd finished, she'd demand money and start to rock the boat or remove the plug. All non-swimmers would pay up right away.

SEX FOR SALE

Two men who mistakenly propositioned an undercover Sydney policewoman told her that they were both keen sociology students and that all they were doing was completing a survey of Australian sex-tariffs.

In October 1994 a thirty-four-year-old Swedish taxi driver had sex with a regular customer in her home on a number of separate occasions and then presented her with a bill for the equivalent of £5,600. Each time they'd had sex, he'd left the meter running.

Prostitutes in Hawaii didn't want a newcomer from Florida muscling into their lucrative trade with wealthy Japanese businessmen, so they decided to sabotage her attempts. The newbie couldn't work out why her advances were spurned – after all she was young and attractive. It wasn't until she was arrested after approaching an undercover officer that the penny dropped. Her so-called hooker friends hadn't been honest when they'd taught her a selection of 'sure-fire' Japanese phrases to attract clients. These included, 'I've got VD. Want to have sex?' and 'Get the fuck out of here, you dirty asshole.'

IS IT IN YET?

In 1994 a Malaysian man took a Kuala Lumpur prostitute back to his hotel room but she became scared when she noticed he had a metal penis that gleamed in the light. She was half right. The man had actually recently undergone a penis-enlargement operation, which involved having ball bearings partially implanted in his penis to give it extra girth. Screaming at this shocking sight, she beat him unconscious, breaking his arm. The man took the prostitute to court for failing to refund his money and for assault. After hearing evidence from both parties – and with the mitigating factor of his unsightly penis – the girl was sentenced to one day in jail.

A case widely reported in the press in 2006 concerns twenty-two-year-old London prostitute Louise Jowett. Arguing over payment while she was having sex with her client Brett O'Leary, she grabbed his penis in her mouth and bit down. He told Ipswich Crown Court, 'She bit hard. She bit very hard. I tried to prise her teeth apart with my fingers. I was pleading with her to stop.'

His ordeal lasted for between thirty and forty-five seconds until Jowett eventually released his penis from her mouth. He noticed he was bleeding heavily. By this point, Jowett had run out of his house and he managed to call the emergency services. 'I was panicking that I was going to bleed to death,' he said.

The jury was told Jowett had bitten Mr O'Leary's penis with such determination that he required surgery to repair it. Such was the force used that, some hours later in hospital, teeth marks could still be seen on the penis.

SEX FOR SALE

When police raided an Irish brothel, they found John Callahan lying naked on a sofa in a state of 'sexual arousal'. Callahan explained to the officers that he was completely innocent of soliciting sex and that – more importantly – he'd had no idea he was actually in a brothel. He explained that he'd 'been brought here by friends to receive treatment for a football injury.'

In February 1990 a customer at a Zimbabwean brothel in Bulawayo was upset and annoyed by the treatment he received. The girls employed had a reputation for mistreating their clients by throwing them out of windows or torturing them with red-hot irons, so he showed his dissatisfaction in the best way he knew: he blew the brothel up with sticks of dynamite, destroying half of its sixty-four rooms.

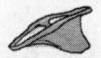

In November 1989 Israeli dentist Jacob Beisvitz of Tel Aviv rang an escort agency but, when the girl arrived at his hotel, he discovered it was his wife Rachel – who quickly left. The couple next saw each other in the divorce court.

Two prostitutes were arrested by Taiwanese police in August 1993. They told the officers they became streetwalkers because they could not resist their sexual urges. Both women were seventy-eight.

IS IT IN YET?

Police were called to a bar in Hermiston, Oregon on a complaint of public indecency. There they found a semi-naked woman about to leave with four men. As officers moved into the arrest, all four of the men protested, claiming that they were the woman's family – specifically, her husband, brother, uncle and cousin – and that all they were doing was giving her a lift home. There was one problem with their story: on further interrogation, none of them knew her name.

The *Vallejo Times-Herald* in Vallejo, California launched a campaign to rid the town of prostitutes, encouraging the police to clean up the local red-light area. Under pressure from the paper, the police successfully did their job. However, the campaign backfired on the newspaper – the hookers relocated in its parking lot.

After collecting money from a bank in Dayton, Ohio, Wells Fargo armoured-car driver Aaron McKie decided to pay for the services of a prostitute and had sex in the vehicle. It was only while he was getting dressed that McKie realised she'd left with a bag containing $80,000.

EXHIBITIONISTS

From the couple who had sex in a photo booth and the soldier directing the traffic with his penis to the man who flashed at department-store mannequins... this section exposes the exposers...

A woman from Entiat, Washington state was sitting in a Laundromat when a man came in and took off all his clothes to wash them. She reported him but sheriff's deputies took no action, stating that the man was from Quebec, 'where such behaviour is not unheard of.'

Michael Monn probably doesn't remember his twenty-third birthday. He broke into a pool bar and, when police found him, they stated he 'had a strong odour of alcohol and was

IS IT IN YET?

semi-incoherent.' They found him naked, his whole body covered in nacho cheese.

In June 1994 two men, aged eighteen and nineteen, who were standing outside Tasty Pizza in Columbia Heights, Minnesota, decided to moon the customers. Upset that no one was taking any notice of their antics, both men began to jump up and down. One of the two lost his balance, fell against the window and smashed it, receiving lacerations to his buttocks and several fingers.

A man in Rothenburg, Germany became a modern-day Humpty Dumpty after climbing to the top of a sixteen-foot-high wall, taking all his clothes off and, to the amusement of passers-by, taking photos of himself. Getting overexcited in the process, he slipped and fell to the garden behind the wall. Fortunately, the only thing hurt was his pride.

Art Prince Jr was caught on video by his neighbour – and subsequently charged with public indecency – semi-naked and having sex with his garden picnic table on four separate occasions. In case you're wondering, he found an unconventional use for the hole where the umbrella usually goes.

EXHIBITIONISTS

In 2005 rugby player Gareth Mason of Aberystwyth, west Wales, who was aged twenty-two, had just returned to his flat from a pub-crawl when he decided to entertain local passers-by from his first-floor window. Dropping his trousers and pants, he stood in the window shouting, 'Who wants some of this?' Unfortunately, he tripped over his trousers and, in front of a friend, fell through the open window on to spiked railings below, bleeding to death after suffering puncture wounds to his neck and chest. An inquest heard how Gareth was found to have a blood-alcohol level four times the drink-drive limit. Flatmate David Wilson said Gareth had tried the stunt before and admitted that people in the house 'occasionally bared their bottoms' to people out of their window.

In July 2009 student Dean Jobling was jailed for thirty-eight weeks for taunting police by simulating sex with an inflatable pig. A court heard that he screamed obscenities at officers outside a pub in Dagenham while gyrating against the pink blow-up toy.

A top freemason lodge master, Malcolm Blaney, faced being expelled from his lodge after exposing himself at a party to celebrate a traditional Masonic village walk. Dressed as a woman, six-foot Blaney took to the dance floor in July 2000 at Lodge 236 in Forth, Lanarkshire, but then lifted his

IS IT IN YET?

dress and flashed onlookers. The *Daily Record* reported that 'Horrified women and men in the audience walked out in disgust.'

One Masonic insider told the newspaper, 'It's the biggest scandal to hit the village in decades. Nobody could believe their eyes.' Someone else commented that Blaney has since been given the nickname Tinky Winky, in tribute to the Teletubbie.

A sixty-five-year-old from Charleswood, Winnipeg was known as the Fence Flasher. His MO was to find a fence panel with a conveniently located knothole and stand behind it with his penis poking through it, thus keeping his identity a secret. Despite being caught on video twice, his identity remains a secret.

Before he was relieved of his duties, a Russian soldier directing traffic at a busy intersection had a novel way to guide traffic left or right. With his trousers round his ankles, he'd hold his penis at the base and wave it energetically back and forth in the direction he wanted the traffic to follow. A witness said that, before long, it was 'as red as a pepper.'

EXHIBITIONISTS

One of the most committed exhibitionists was a man who would masturbate in a south London public phone box during a particularly cold spell in the winter of 1985. Several women reported him exposing himself when it was seven degrees below freezing.

In 1996 a Burbank couple – Melvin Hoffman, fifty-three, and Regina Chatien, forty-three – were found guilty of lewd conduct after being witnessed by an off-duty policeman engaging in oral sex in the stand during an LA Dodgers game the previous summer. They were sentenced to 120 hours' community service, having to buy one hundred tickets for Dodgers' games for charity and to stay away from the Stadium while on probation. The Deputy City Attorney commented that what made it particularly offensive was that the couple's four children – aged between eight and fourteen – were in close proximity.

A man from Edmonton, north London was charged with sending obscene material via the Royal Mail after a local woman received Polaroids of his genitals. She had no trouble in tracking him down, as he'd written his name and address on the back. In his defence, the man claimed they were meant for a sex-contact magazine but that he'd got the addresses mixed up.

IS IT IN YET?

A forty-seven-year-old Dallas flasher, known only as Richard, would stand naked by a railroad bridge and expose himself to passing motorists. When police officers were called, he was having a break, still naked. On seeing them approach, he grabbed his clothes and leaped from the bridge, missing his intended target – a concrete support underneath – and, instead, plummeted thirty-five feet to the ground. He died in nearby Parkland Hospital later that day.

In the old Abcat porn cinema on the Caledonian Road in King's Cross, there was an accepted unwritten code of behaviour that meant, if you sat in the first row, you could masturbate with your penis in your trousers, while sitting in the second row and behind meant you could take it out.

When police arrested David Sorg, twenty-nine, of St Petersburg, Florida for exposing himself in public, he offered the excuse that he used to be a male stripper and he 'missed the attention he got on stage.'

In 1980 a flasher exposed himself to Julie Barlow – a student at the University of Chicago – and asked, 'What do you think of this then?' Miss Barlow studied him for a moment and then declared, 'It looks like a cock to me... only smaller.'

EXHIBITIONISTS

On responding to complaints from customers at a Laundromat, police from Hancock, Michigan found a naked man playing the accordion. The man – a Brazilian graduate student – told officers, 'I can't play the accordion unless I am completely nude.'

To stripper Margaret Cooper, it was just 'another job'. She was briefed to turn up dressed as a police officer and then 'arrest' an elderly man, tie him to his chair, remove his trousers and strip down to her G-string in front of him – all routine for her. Caught up in her performance, however, she failed to realise until it was too late that the man she was now standing almost naked in front of was, in fact, her grandfather.

A fifty-year-old man, known only as 'Gypsy Joe', appeared at Shepton Mallet court in July 1992 to answer a charge of 'lewdly exposing himself to women'. No sooner had the man been asked if he understood the charge than he flashed the three magistrates and then the public gallery.

In 1984 Edwin Johnson strolled down London's Charing Cross Road and, in quick succession, exposed himself to two men, a teenage girl and then two plainclothes policemen,

IS IT IN YET?

who duly arrested him. What was odd about the incident, however, was that Johnson had no penis. He was in the process of a sex-change operation and also went by the name Linda Gold. As women can't be charged with indecent exposure, Johnson/Gold was, instead, charged with insulting behaviour. When asked if he had anything to say, he flashed the station sergeant.

A science lecturer from Cambridge, Massachusetts was accused of indecent exposure by one of his students but he explained in court that it was completely unintentional. His excuse was that his washing machine was defective and left soap powder on his clothes, to which he was allergic. To alleviate the rash on his genitals, he said, he would poke his penis through his underwear. He explained that, during a tutorial with the student in question, he unfortunately caught a whiff of her perfume and this caused him to have an erection. He told the court, 'Even more unfortunately, I had unwittingly left open my fly and my erection poked through my lab coat – and here I am.'

He was cleared of all charges.

Californian police arrested a flasher in a department store, although none of his victims would press charges. That's because the flasher in question was exposing himself to the display mannequins before fondling them. Commenting on

EXHIBITIONISTS

the unusual crime, a police officer said, 'I hope this is the first of a series of none.'

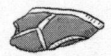

A couple were seen entering a photo booth together at Portsmouth Central Station, where they were later arrested for trying to sell pictures to commuters of themselves committing a sex act. At court, it transpired that they had just met fifteen minutes before the photographs were taken and that she'd done it as she needed the money for a ticket to Haslemere to see her boyfriend.

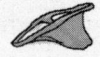

An eighteen-year-old exhibitionist from Ljungby in southern Sweden thought he could remain anonymous after setting up a number of fake Facebook accounts and sending photos of his genitals to a series of women, many of whom were old school friends. He was tracked down and arrested in May 2014 after one of his victims recognised the distinctive wallpaper behind him in the shots, since it matched wallpaper seen in an Instagram post. She made the connection between the two accounts, which led to the man being prosecuted for sexual harassment and being ordered to pay 5,000 kronor in damages.

IS IT IN YET?

In November 2013 fifty-one-year-old David Sherratt walked into the bar of his local, the White Hart, in Tunstall, Stoke-on-Trent, Staffs, naked from the waist down and carrying a bag of sex toys. He then proceeded to challenge anyone who was unhappy with his lack of clothing to go outside to settle the problem. At his subsequent court appearance, he admitted causing harassment, alarm and distress and was handed a twelve-month community order.

A freezing New York winter didn't prevent a flasher from going about his business. However, instead of exposing himself in the flesh, he would whip out photos showing his erect penis. The NYPD commented, 'He probably felt he couldn't measure up in the cold. We've never heard of this before. People are still shocked.'

In May 2012 a flasher ran into a bookshop in Newtown, Philadelphia and, according to a report, 'whipped out his junk then ran away.' What he didn't realise was that it was a specialist bookshop for the blind.

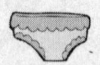

A couple in Washington DC decided to add spice to their sex lives by indulging in some oral sex when out for a romantic dinner. Concealed by the table, the women went down on

EXHIBITIONISTS

her partner but suffered an epileptic fit in the middle and suddenly bit down on his penis. Acting on reflex, he grabbed his fork and stabbed her in the head so she'd release him. Both were admitted to a local hospital.

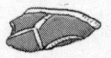

Seattle resident Vladimir Mishkov, twenty-six, couldn't stop exposing himself. In June 2012 he was on his way from prison to court to face a flashing charge, when he couldn't resist the opportunity to expose his genitals to a prison employee.

Australian serial flasher Clifford John Candy, thirty, who had exposed himself in public nineteen times over a decade, explained to a Brisbane judge in June 2012 that he had a rational reason as to why he liked to wave his genitals around 'like a flag'. It was to overcome his fear of being naked in public.

In 2007 an Israeli couple were ticketed for having sex in their car. Their act was brought to the attention of the police since they failed to pull in to a quiet and discreet side road – deciding, instead, to have sex in the middle of traffic while frustrated drivers had to swerve around their stationary car.

OUCH!

Incidents involving severed penises, torn-off testicles and a chilli in the vagina. Plus, of course, how that accident with the vacuum cleaner happened while vacuuming the house in the nude...

After a drunken row at their home in Frankfurt-an-der-Oder, Heidi Siebe cut off her boyfriend's penis with a breadknife. She said that she did it because Hans-Joachim Kampioni (fifty-six) always pestered her for sex. She knocked him out with a stool before going to work with the knife, then tried to cover her tracks by setting fire to the house. The penis was damaged in the blaze and could not be reattached, so Kampioni auctioned it at his local pub, where it raised the equivalent of £40 and bottle of schnapps. He told patrons there, 'It's no use to me anymore.'

IS IT IN YET?

Ronald Elmore arrived at the ER at the Bossier Medical Center in Louisiana with both his testicles cut off. He told staff that he'd met a woman at a bar, taken her home and that she'd castrated him while he slept. Later on, he changed his story and told them that he and his wife had been taking drugs and that, when he found himself impotent, he told her to castrate him. Finally, Elmore told the truth. He said he'd castrated himself for the hell of it and put his testicles in his freezer, where police later found them.

Twenty-four-year-old Amanda Monti of Birkenhead, Merseyside had split up with her lover Geoffrey Jones but stayed on good terms with him. In May 2004 she picked him up from a party and went back to his house with a few friends for drinks. There she offered him sex but, when Jones refused, she flew into a rage, grabbing his crotch and tearing off his left testicle with her bare hands. She then tried to swallow it before spitting it out. A friend at the party then handed it back to Jones, saying, 'That's yours.' At her trial at Liverpool Crown Court in January 2005, Monti admitted wounding and was jailed for two-and-a-half years. She told the court, 'I am in no way a violent person.'

A nursing journal reports these excuses given to doctors on duty at A&E wards as to why victims injured their penises in accidents involving vacuum cleaners:

OUCH!

- 'I was experimenting with nudism. While cleaning the house, I was trying to vacuum a cobweb off the ceiling when I slipped and the nozzle "grabbed" the lightest of my body extensions.'
- 'I was sitting down with the nozzle between my legs, trying to clear a blockage. I did this successfully but forgot I'd not switched off the cleaner.'
- 'I was vacuuming a friend's staircase wearing a loose-fitting dressing gown when I leaned across to unplug it. At that point, the dressing gown came undone and my penis was sucked into the vacuum cleaner.'
- 'I was told that this was a way to reduce water retention.'
- 'I was changing the plug in the nude when it accidentally turned itself on.'
- 'I couldn't afford the course of liposuction, so I tried a "do it yourself" treatment.'

According to a report in the *Calgary Sun*, thirty-five-year-old Gerald Allan Naud — a former professional boxer from Edmonton, Canada — admitted harassing women to kick him in the balls. Detective Wil Tonowski stated, 'This offender has a history of asking women to kick him between the legs because of a $50 bet he's made with his buddies,' adding, 'But there are no buddies… the guy is a masochist.'

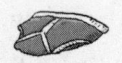

IS IT IN YET?

A highly agitated Norwich woman visited her local GP, sweating profusely, refusing to sit down in the reception area. When it was her turn to see the doctor, she still refused to sit down and blurted out that she had a chilli in her vagina. When the GP asked if it was stuck, she said, 'No. I just want some advice.' Thinking on his feet, the GP replied, 'Well, my advice is take it out of your vagina and never put it back in again.' When he asked the woman if she'd like to tell him why she had a chilli up there in the first place, she calmly replied, 'No, thanks. You've been a lot of help already,' and just left.

A man complaining of acute genital pain had to admit to doctors that, while engaging in sex with his wife about twelve years earlier, he'd let her insert a mascara brush into his penis. X-rays revealed that the top of the brush had broken off and that fibrous tissue had grown around it – the cause of the severe pain.

In 2004 sixty-seven-year-old Constantin Mocanu, from a village near the south-eastern town of Galati in Bulgaria, rushed out into his yard in his underwear to kill a noisy chicken that had been keeping him awake at night. However, according to the state Rompres news agency, in the darkness, he accidentally cut off his penis. Mr Mocanu is quoted as saying, 'I confused it with the chicken's neck. I cut it … and the dog rushed and ate it.' He was admitted to the emergency hospital in Galati, bleeding heavily, but survived his ordeal.

In 2002 a Romanian couple from Craiova ended up in their local A&E after a kitchen frolic got out of hand. It started when the man was cooking pancakes and his girlfriend decided to strip and perform oral sex on him. Momentarily losing his concentration, the man accidentally spilled hot oil on his girlfriend's back. This caused her to, first, instinctively bite down hard and then thrust her head back, cracking it on the frying pan. The man was treated for lacerations to his penis, while his girlfriend suffered burns to her back and a cut scalp.

A Leicester man who complained about severe stomach pains was found to have an acupuncture needle in his bladder. When questioned about how it had got there, the man admitted that he'd inserted it into his penis. When asked why, he told the doctor, 'For fun.'

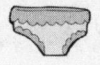

Although there are no actual bones in the penis, it is possible for the fibrous tubes that fill with blood during an erection to break. This usually happens when an erect penis is forcefully bent – an act usually accompanied by a loud

IS IT IN YET?

snapping sound and agonising pain. One man in his sixties reportedly suffered a penile fracture when he was manically masturbating and, hearing his elderly mother approaching his bedroom, attempted to quickly lock the door. In his panic, he slipped and fell down directly on his penis.

Similarly, a thirty-eight-year-old Essex man was attempting to have sex with his wife Anna when he missed the target and, instead, hit her pelvis, suffering a similar fracture. His wife summed it up perfectly when she said, 'We were having sex and he missed and broke his willy.'

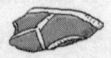

A couple accidently spiced up their sex life when the man came home from a night out and decided to go down on his wife, forgetting that he'd previously eaten a really hot curry. The intense burning sensation usually experienced from a curry is due to the sensitive mucous membrane that lines our mouths – the same membrane that also lines the vagina. His wife screamed in agony after he inadvertently burned her 'sensitive lady parts'.

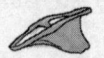

In his book *Hollywood Babylon*, author Kenneth Anger claimed that actor James Dean was sexually excited by pain. He allegedly had a thing for being kicked and beaten and liked to have cigarettes put out on his bare chest. His nickname was 'The Human Ashtray'.

OUCH!

The Ponapeans of the Eastern Caroline Islands in the Pacific Ocean find that an enlarged labia and clitoris are sexually attractive, so much so that the women apply stinging ants to their genitals in order to cause swelling.

In March 2013 Sharai Mawera was having sex with her boyfriend in a secluded spot in the bush in the northern town of Kariba in Zimbabwe when they were interrupted by a loud roar. Unfortunately, this wasn't a cry of passion from her unidentified lover but the sound of a lion. Ignoring any thoughts of gallantry, her boyfriend ran off naked to raise the alarm but, by the time help had arrived, Sharai had been mauled to death.

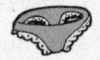

Pioneering sexologist Alfred Kinsey had erotic secrets of his own. A 1997 biography revealed for the first time that, as a teenager, he would insert a straw into his penis, before progressing to pipe cleaners and then, in later life, a toothbrush – bristles first – to provoke ejaculation.

Thirty-year-old Sergei Abramov was so sick and tired of his wife mocking his ability to maintain an erection that he decided to do something about it. Eschewing seeking medical advice, he decided to keep his penis rigid by inserting a thermometer into it. The sex session was agonisingly cut short when the end of the thermometer painfully slipped into and injured his bladder.

Tamakeri (Japanese for 'ball kicking') is a sexual fetish and sub-genre of pornography, in which a man's testicles are abused. Originally just popular in Japan, this genre now has worldwide appeal.

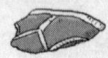

A Thai woman, jealous of her philandering husband, attacked him with scissors, snipped off his penis and threw it out of her apartment window. The man could only look on in shock as he saw a duck waddle off with his penis in its mouth.

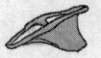

In some Arab cultures, circumcision didn't just mean removing the foreskin; the penis was stripped of a layer of flesh along its whole length. Tradition stated that, if the boy cried out, it meant he was unworthy of manhood and his father would be permitted to kill him. It has been reported that one in five boys died this way.

OUCH!

According to the Old Testament (1 Samuel 18:27), King Saul of the Hebrews told David that he could only marry his daughter Michal if he could present a hundred foreskins removed from slain Philistine warriors. To impress his future father-in-law, David returned with twice the required amount.

Suffering from Peyronie's disease is enough to send you round the bend. Those afflicted by this condition (estimated at about 5 per cent of men) find their penis turning into the shape of a boomerang, making intercourse not just difficult but extremely painful. The change in shape occurs when a fibrous area on the penis contracts, slowly drawing the penis to that side. There is no cure for the condition. However, surgical correction is possible but is highly specialised. Since one of the consequences is penile shortening, many sufferers decline this operation.

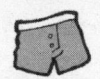

In December 1994 shoplifter Barry Quem – a twenty-five-year-old from Boston – attempted to steal five live lobsters from a local supermarket by stuffing them down his underpants. Police were alerted to the theft when Barry began screaming as soon as he left the supermarket – one of the lobsters had tightened its claw around his penis. He was rushed to a nearby ER and the claw was eventually removed with pliers. The doctor who examined him stated that Barry had effectively performed a 'do-it-yourself vasectomy.'

IS IT IN YET?

The emergency services were horrified to hear how a New Jersey man had been stabbed in his genitals by a complete stranger who'd got into his bed. It wasn't long, however, before the truth came out. The reality was that he'd attempted to have sex with his vacuum cleaner, severing the tip of his penis in the process.

BE SATISFIED WITH WHAT GOD GAVE YOU

'It's not how long it is, it's what you do with it.' Try telling that to the men who suffered botched enlargement operations or who injected their penises with everything from horse drugs to hair tonic to make them more impressive, with the inevitable catastrophic results…

In May 2011 a New Jersey woman, Kasia Rivera, was arrested on manslaughter charges after a DIY penis enlargement went wrong, causing the death of twenty-two-year-old Justin Street. Ignoring the fact that the substance was used as an aid to enlarging breasts rather than penises, Ms Rivera injected silicone into Mr Street's manhood. The result was his death the next day from a blood clot.

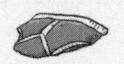

IS IT IN YET?

In 2007 a Malaysian man was hospitalised after getting a large, heavy nut (the non-food type) stuck firmly around his penis. The Kuala-Lumpur resident – a welder by trade – explained to doctors that he'd hoped the heavy weight would stretch his penis because he was desperate to impress his girlfriend.

Since he received a penis pump as a present when he was twenty, Micha Stunz (now forty-five) from Berlin has always wanted to modify his manhood. He started to inject his penis with saline solution but stopped after becoming aware of the risk of infection and the fact that the effect was only temporary. He then met a medical student who agreed to inject his penis and scrotum with silicone. The result is an unfeasibly large penis nine inches long and three-and-a-half inches wide (not circumference) that weighs half a stone. The use of silicone can still lead to infection of the penis. However, Micha told *vice.com* that he is aware of the risks. As a result of the injections, he can't get a visible erection and said he had to be 'more inventive' in the bedroom. He commented, 'After you reach a certain size, you can't do certain things any more.'

Paramedics called to a disco in Salt Lake City, Utah found a young man collapsed on the floor. Witnesses said that one minute he was happily dancing and the next he was on the floor turning blue. The paramedics identified that the man

BE SATISFIED WITH WHAT GOD GAVE YOU

had suffered a heart attack but he died in the ambulance before reaching hospital. Later examination revealed the exact cause. To impress girls at the disco, he'd strapped a roll of quarters to his crotch, tying them tightly with a roll of surgical tape. This cut off the circulation to his leg and it was this lack of blood flow combined with the energetic dancing that had triggered the heart attack.

A Guyana newspaper carried the report of a man who, wishing to impress his new girlfriend, injected himself with Cantarden, a drug used to put horses in heat. The drug had its desired effect: a huge erection that was both painful and incessant. After a few days of agony, the man sought medical advice and eventually underwent surgery to reverse the condition. Unfortunately, a side effect was an inability to get another erection.

A large number of American men responded to an ad promoting what they thought was the bargain of the century: a penis enlarger for only $25. All, however, was not how it seemed. They were all very disappointed (and too embarrassed to complain) when the only thing they received was a magnifying glass.

IS IT IN YET?

'Botched operation' are two words no one wants to hear. Add the words 'penis enlargement' in the middle and you know the story involves a whole world of pain. It happened to a Philadelphia resident in 1998. Known only as 'John', he told reporters, 'I was an average-sized guy but any man's ego tells him whatever he's got isn't enough.' He visited a specialist and underwent the $6,000 operation in New York. Two weeks after the operation, which involved cutting ligaments and injecting fat into his penis, he knew things weren't right. He was in considerable pain and a second surgical procedure only made it worse. The end result was that his penis became infected and the skin fell off, and most of it had to be cut away.

John was left with a penis about an inch-and-a-half long and is also impotent. Remaining stoic, however, he commented, 'Though it's good to pee out of.'

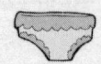

According to the *Bangkok Post*, at least a hundred men in Thailand underwent bogus penis-enlargement operations. The paper reported that the doctors who performed the surgery injected the men's penises with a mixture of olive oil, chalk and other unknown substances to provide bulk. An official at a hospital in Chiang Mai told the paper, 'I've even seen penises containing bits of the Bangkok telephone directory.'

BE SATISFIED WITH WHAT GOD GAVE YOU

From the onset of puberty, members form the Karamojong tribe in north-eastern Uganda tie stones to the tips of their penises in order to elongate them. By the time the boy has reached his late teens years, he may be carrying up to 20 lbs on his penis. Eventually, the organs become so stretched that, in order to better manage their rather impractical appendages, the Karamojong tie their penises in knots and tuck them away.

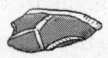

In October 2010 Michael D. Nash, sixty-one, underwent penile-implant surgery at the Veterans Administration Hospital in Lexington, Kentucky and left with his penis amputated. His $10-million lawsuit launched against the hospital alleges that a nurse put an ice pack on his penis to ease the swelling in post-op and left it there for nineteen hours straight, rather than removing it after two to four hours. As a result, Nash's penis developed frostbite and gangrene. His lawyer, Lawrence Jones, stated that amputation was required after his client had been left with 'this dark, black rotting piece of the most important part of the body,' and added that Nash was planning to undergo reconstructive surgery.

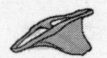

In November 2012 a fifty-year-old man was admitted to the Police General Hospital in Bangkok after his penis had swelled to the size of a coconut. According to the *Bangkok Post*, the man had been to an illegal clinic for a penis-enlargement operation, during which his penis was injected with olive oil. The swelling was the result of a cancerous infection and doctors had no choice but to remove his penis.

Sixty-year-old Miami resident Enrique Milla underwent penile-implant surgery in 2007 to correct erectile dysfunction but lost his penis to flesh-eating bacteria nine days later, according to the report by Courthouse News Service. He settled out of court with the urologist who performed the operation.

A man who wished to remain nameless went to Turkey to have a sophisticated penile implant fitted, only to discover a big problem when he arrived back home on Merseyside. This particular implant was operated by a remote control – and the man discovered it shared the same frequency as his neighbour's garage door. This meant he got an erection – or lost it – at completely random and, sometimes, very inopportune times. According to the man, doctors will not help him because the alleged medical negligence happened in Turkey with equipment not recognised in the UK. Talking about his neighbour, he commented, 'Every time his car pulls in, I can't leave the house.'

BE SATISFIED WITH WHAT GOD GAVE YOU

A thirty-five-year-old Cambodian man thought that anything that made his hair grow longer would have the same effect on his penis – so in June 2007 he injected his manhood with hair tonic. The resultant and consistent pain was so intense that the man ended up hanging himself to relieve the agony. Although the death was deemed a suicide, details were released to the newspapers, so that the use of these sort of home remedies should serve as a warning to other Cambodians not to try this at home. Coroner Vieng Vannarith commented, 'He wanted a bigger one very badly and the results were tragic.'

A fifty-two-year-old Turkish man tried to persuade doctors to replace his own penis with one he'd removed from a donkey. The story came to light when the man was shot and injured by his son in an attempt to get him to stop obsessing about this operation.

It was reported in July 2014 that an anonymous Australian, known only as Mike, remortgaged his home in order to raise A$50,000 to fund a second penis enlargement operation. Thirty-two-year-old builder Mike has a penis that was just 7 cm long when erect and suffers from low self-esteem and depression. The first round of surgery cost A$45,000 and was unsuccessful; complications made his penis even smaller.

PLAYING AWAY

Hell hath no fury like a woman scorned... That's why one man discovered, too late, that his wife had put pepper spray in his condoms, another man had his penis super-glued to his stomach, while another had his penis cut off and tied to a helium balloon (and no, he didn't get it back)...

An Austrian woman was having an affair with a cartoonist and, for a laugh, he decided to draw a small cartoon on one of her buttocks. Unfortunately, the woman forgot to wash it off and, when she undressed that night in front of her husband, he not only saw the cartoon but he knew right away who'd drawn it – the cartoonist in question had carefully signed his work.

IS IT IN YET?

In 1994, after Boris Paveharik of Poland had sex with his mistress, he was rushed to hospital in incredible pain, suffering from severe penile inflammation. Unbeknown to him, his wife had previously discovered a packet of condoms in his pocket and had carefully injected them with pepper spray.

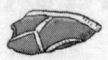

A Mexican man, known only as Esteban, had a peculiar quirk: he could only make love to his wife if he heard strident marching music. His wife Anna became suspicious when he began to take his gramophone with him on business trips, so she hired a private detective to investigate. The two of them followed him to a hotel and waited silently outside his room. As soon as they heard a loud march strike up, they burst in and caught Esteban naked with his mistress.

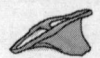

Coming home unexpectedly, a Rio de Janeiro husband found his wife in bed with her lover. Drawing a gun on the couple, he decided to teach them a lesson and made his wife super-glue her hand on to the man's penis. The lovers were successfully separated after surgery but the man died, subsequently, from toxins in the glue. As a result, the husband was charged with murder.

PLAYING AWAY

A similar incident took place in Harrisburg, Pennsylvania. After discovering that her boyfriend had been seeing another girl, a sixteen-year-old took her revenge by getting him into a state of excitement and then, when his eyes were closed as he savoured the moment, super-gluing his penis to his stomach.

In Singapore a man who suspected his wife of having an affair hired a private eye to follow her. He was right. The detective was observing the woman giving her boss a blow job in his parked car when he suddenly witnessed something a lot more dramatic. A van accidentally rammed into the car and the force of the collision caused her to bite off his penis. The detective later commented, 'There was a loud scream from the woman whose mouth was covered with blood.' Nobly, he ceased his surveillance and called an ambulance to take the injured man to hospital.

On discovering that forty-seven-year-old Prayoon Eklang was having an affair, a jealous Thai wife drugged him and then cut off his penis while he was asleep. To add insult to injury, she then tied it to a helium balloon and let it go.

IS IT IN YET?

When Chris Taylor's African Grey parrot Ziggy kept mimicking kissing noises every time it heard the name Gary on TV or the radio, Chris dismissed it as just a funny quirk. The cat was well and truly out of the bag, however, when he snuggled next to his girlfriend Suzy in their Leeds flat and Ziggy cried out in her voice, 'I love you Gary!'

Suzy broke down in tears and confessed she'd been having a four-month fling with a former colleague. She'd met her lover in the flat several times and Ziggy had witnessed everything. Chris and Suzy split up and Chris had to get Ziggy re-homed. He commented: 'I wasn't sorry to see the back of Suzy after what she did, but it really broke my heart to let Ziggy go. I love him to bits and I really miss having him around, but it was torture hearing him repeat that name over and over again.'

An Australian woman awoke one night to hear sounds of heavy breathing from the garden. She looked out of her window and saw her husband having sex in the flowerbed with a complete stranger. His defence was that he suffered from 'sexsomnia': a condition whereby the sufferer is compelled to commit sexual acts in their sleep.

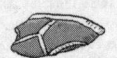

In September 2002 Jorge Armando Flores was having sex with his girlfriend when she whispered in his ear that, in order to fulfil one of her long-held sexual fantasies, he first had to close his eyes. Wondering what pleasures awaited, Flores dutifully complied, only for his girlfriend to knife him in the neck and chest. She then called the police to admit what she'd done and Flores was rushed to hospital, where he recovered from his injuries. The girlfriend told the authorities that the reason she stabbed him was because, when they made love, he always called out the name of his ex-girlfriend.

While having sex with his mistress in his car, a Finnish man accidentally hit a speed-dial button on his mobile phone – the button assigned to his wife. When she answered the call, all she could hear was a strange female voice shouting passionately, 'I love you.' What's more, she recognised the voice as belonging to a close friend. Later that evening, she went round to the friend's house and, without warning, punched her in the face. She was later charged with assault. The state of the marriage was not recorded.

YOU'RE NICKED!

There's a saying, 'Don't do the crime if you can't do the time.' After considering the following incidents, like the man who tried to smuggle cocaine in an unbelievably oversize fake penis, the man who performed a sexual act with a stuffed toy in a crowded supermarket or the lovers who had sex on the bonnet of a police patrol car, there should also be a new adage: 'Don't do the crime if you're a fucking idiot.'

An Australian thief walked into a Sydney sex shop and threatened staff with a baseball bat unless they handed him cash from the till. He was soon caught by police. While he was waiting for the money, he thumbed through a porno mag, leaving his incriminating fingerprints behind.

IS IT IN YET?

Police in the town of Cook, Australia arrested Thomas Borkman, twenty-four, for breaking into the apartment of a random thirty-one-year-old woman and super-gluing his face to the sole of her foot while she slept. The two were separated after a three-hour procedure and police speculated that Borkman's bizarre act 'had some sexual significance.'

In 2012 a man was arrested in Harvard, Idaho and charged with indecent exposure. He'd been seen waving his penis at a dog.

A huge bulge in a man's trousers attracted the attention of most of the guests in a Dubai bar, including an off-duty policeman, who couldn't – or didn't want to – believe anyone could be that well-endowed. Acting on just a gut feel, the policeman frisked the man and his hunch was correct. He was found to be wearing a fake penis, filled to the brim with cocaine.

A similar incident involved a would-be American drugs smuggler. To stash his heroin, he created a realistic-looking fake penis to fool any customs inspections. He was caught out for three reasons: a) it was far too pink, b) it was eight inches long flaccid and c) the real giveaway… at the inspection, it became detached.

YOU'RE NICKED!

Police in Stevens Point, Wisconsin arrested Della Dobbs, thirty-one, for theft. Her MO was to meet men in bars and offer to take them to her pick-up truck for sex. Before beginning, however, she told them to undress and roll around in the snow to get more sexually excited. While they were following her advice, she'd drive off with their wallets.

Retired grocer Donald James Brown of Colorado Springs would cut pictures of people from the local newspaper and superimpose their heads on photos from porno mags. He'd then send the photos to the people and threaten to kidnap them and make them perform oral sex acts. He was tracked by police after he'd sent threats to thirty-nine people.

In February 2002 police in Dacula, Georgia arrested a twenty-two-year-old man in a pumpkin patch after a passing patrol car spotted him having 'intimate relations' with a piece of fruit, in which he'd cut a small hole. After his arrest, the man gave a phone interview to reporters from the Gwinett County Jail to explain his actions, saying, 'You know, a pumpkin is soft and squishy inside and there was no one around here for miles,' before adding, 'At least, I thought there wasn't.'

IS IT IN YET?

In 2005 a twenty-five-year-old Australian man with a grudge against the police decided to show his contempt for the law keepers by masturbating over a parked police cruiser. The mistake he made was that the car was right in front of the police station and in full view of the officers working there.

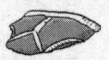

In July 2014 police arrested Takahiko Naito and Atsuko Sonoda, in Kyoto, Japan for selling shoes fitted with miniature cameras designed for filming women's underwear. So-called 'upskirt photos' are very popular in Japan, with millions searching for images online. The two men were charged with assisting in causing a public nuisance. The cameras were sold between October 2013 and March 2014, with the photos being taken by a remote control concealed in the pocket. Police became aware of the shoes after one of the buyers was arrested for taking upskirt photos of a schoolgirl. After his arrest, Sonoda told police he didn't know what customers were going to do with the cameras.

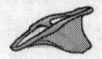

Learning of his infidelity, Francisca Vega of Barcelona poisoned her husband Javier and, using a process developed by a research chemist who studied a tribe of head-hunters in Borneo, shrunk his naked body down to the size of a doll and kept the body pickled in formaldehyde in a jar in her pantry. The police inspector on the case commented on the husband's body, 'He was sitting in this jar with his head tilted back and his mouth wide open. He looked like a fat little baby with a man's face.' Francisca spent a year in a mental hospital before being released.

Chiu Yu-kit — a thirty-one-year-old Hong Kong Television Reporter at Asia Television (ATV) — was arrested for masturbating naked on the top deck of a bus. At his trial in September 2008, Yu-kit pleaded guilty to one count of indecency in public. The court heard that an off-duty police officer made the arrest after he jogged past the bus, looked up and saw the reporter standing on a seat naked and facing a window. Yu-kit explained that he had committed the act to relieve stress. Passing a one-year suspended sentence, the judge advised Yu-kit to exercise or talk to others if he wanted to relax.

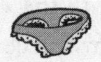

In September 2006 a sixty-nine-year-old man from Huntington Beach, California was arrested on four misdemeanour changes, including animal cruelty. According to the police report, he'd broken into La Purisima Mission Park, then stripped naked, rolled around in the dirt and then covered himself in olive oil and oats so nearby horses would 'lick him clean.' Deputies said he had driven to Lompoc from Huntington Beach specifically for the purpose of fulfilling his fantasy. They added that it did not appear that any animal was injured.

IS IT IN YET?

According to the *Mainichi Daily News*, in January 2006 Masafumi Natsukawa, thirty-nine, was arrested in Yokohama, Japan for allegedly tricking more than thirty young girls to open their mouths on the pretence that he was checking for tooth decay. When they opened wide, he licked their tongues.

In October 2014 nineteen-year-old Sean Johnson was arrested after being caught on camera in his local Walmart store performing 'a solo sex act' with a stuffed animal and then returning it in a polluted state to the shelf, before fleeing. The incident was captured by security cameras in the store in Brooksville, Florida. According to local news channel WFLA, Johnson later confessed to police and was charged with indecent exposure. The store declared any products that had come into contact with the stuffed toy as 'contaminated' and they were removed from sale.

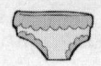

An Italian farmhand from Biassa in Italy was arrested in August 1988 for dancing naked in a local cemetery – a daily practice. At his court appearance, he had to be protected from angry widows who he'd upset by his antics. In his defence, he claimed the naked cemetery dancing was the only pleasure he had in life.

YOU'RE NICKED!

A horny couple in Groningen, Holland were having sex on the bonnet of a parked car when they were arrested. The lovers were so engrossed in their act that they failed to realise that the bonnet in question belonged to a police patrol car.

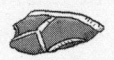

Joseph Silvertsen and his girlfriend were having sex in an alley in Spenard, Alaska in June 2002, when pedestrian Jerome King spotted them and asked, 'Are you having fun?' Mr Silvertsen took offence to this interruption and chased Mr King, picking up a two-foot-long piece of pipe on the way and hitting King repeatedly. Silvertsen was later arrested on a second-degree assault charge. The *Anchorage Daily News* commented, 'Spontaneous interruption of a public sex act to engage in an aggravated assault should be considered as a strong indication of a seriously unaddressed anger-management problem.'

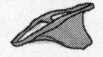

A thirty-four-year-old teacher was arrested in Clydebank, Scotland after he was seen sitting in his parked car, pleasuring himself with a vibrator that was being powered from his cigarette lighter.

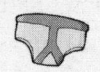

IS IT IN YET?

Patricia Orionno of the French town of Doubs could not put up with her husband Jean-Louis's constant pestering for sex several times a day, so in 1988 she tried to kill him. An overdose of sleeping tablets ground up in a meat pie just made him oversleep, so she then resorted to trying to cut his wrists, gassing him and then suffocating him with a pillow. When none of these worked, she stabbed him in the chest eight times. She was charged with murder but was later acquitted, as this was deemed a crime of passion.

Fifty-nine-year-old Roger Powell of Enfield, North Carolina was arrested in May 2000 after a boy saw him having sex with a pig in nearby woods. According to the police, Powell was talking to the pig while taking part in the act. The accused explained that he'd been having relations with pigs at least twice a day for a year because he didn't want to catch any diseases from his girlfriend, who he labelled a 'crack whore'. Powell was subsequently charged with a crime against nature – a felony in North Carolina.

Hungarian policewoman Livia Kovacs was sacked after being spotted by colleagues in an S&M dominatrix movie; not because she appeared in the film but because she was wearing her regulation uniform and using police-issue handcuffs.

YOU'RE NICKED!

Police stopping random vehicles as part of a drink-driving clampdown in the Ibiza resort of Playa d'en Bosa were surprised to discover three couples having an orgy in the back of a van. However, instead of being charged with public indecency, the six Swiss nationals were fined €200 for not wearing seat belts.

A twenty-three-year-old computer-engineering student at Fresno State University, California admitted having sex with a sheep on campus because he was 'stressed'. He stated that he'd gone to the university's barn after a night of heavy drinking because he had an important exam coming up. He'd intended to take out his frustrations by 'beating up some cows' but was overheard by classmates, who tipped off the police. When they arrived, they found him on top of the sheep with his trousers around his ankles. When arrested, the student's only comment was, 'Am I going to be expelled for this?'

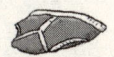

In 2014 Edwin Tobergta, thirty-five, was arrested for having sex with an inflatable Li-lo on a public road in Hamilton, Ohio – but it wasn't his first offence. In fact, he has a history of sexual encounters with plastic air mattresses. In 2013 he was jailed for eleven months for outraging public decency, while in 2002 he was caught having sex with an inflatable pumpkin that was part of a neighbour's Halloween display. When Tobergta appeared in court for his latest offence, he wore a T-shirt that said, appropriately enough, 'I'm out of my mind. Please leave a message.'

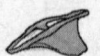

A seventy-six-year-old woman from Crown Point, Indiana called police after she awoke to find a strange man tickling her feet. When police arrived, the man was still in her house and was immediately arrested. He admitted breaking in but told police he was 'just looking for water.'

Charles Cook of Weymouth was a serious leg fetishist who was arrested in 1980 for perpetrating a rather sad scam. He would writhe on the floor pretending to have broken his arm, just so he could look up the skirts of any sympathetic passers-by who came to help him.

A man arrested for taking secret photographs of 'man-boobs' at a swimming pool had the case against him dismissed after the court of appeal ruled that, under the 2003 Sexual Offences Act, only women's breasts can be considered 'sexual'.

THAT'S JUST WRONG!

When it comes to sexual acts, who's to say what's right and what's wrong? Well, call me old fashioned but having sex with a statue, road signs, a scarecrow, a teddy bear, the pavement, a shoe, metal railings, a corpse and a cow's heart... now that's just wrong!

In June 1991 Mervyn Lilburne, thirty-nine, of Ballarat, Australia was fined the equivalent of £200 for obscene exposure and criminal damage in a local park. He'd been caught trying to have sex with a statue. The damage happened when he was surprised and fell into a flowerbed.

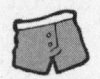

In 2007 Ron Baxter from Sioux Falls, South Dakota was arrested by police after they observed him simulating sex

IS IT IN YET?

with a 'Stop' sign. A search of his home revealed a collection of videos of him masturbating with various traffic signs.

Closer to home, in March 2008 an anonymous thirty-two-year-old man from Wiltshire was charged with 'simulating a sex act with a lamp post.' According to news reports, this incident was the latest in a spate of bizarre sex crimes in the area involving inanimate objects.

What's worse than capturing stray cats and then ritually stabbing them in the heart? Masturbating the instant they die. Russian police caught a fourteen-year-old Russian boy doing just that and discovered a whole 'cat cemetery' in his garden, containing over thirty animals.

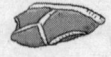

In 1995 it was reported that a teenager from Knoxville, Tennessee was found dead in his bedroom after firefighters were called to his family home by neighbours who smelled burning. According to authorities, the house was empty apart from the boy, who was found nude, with the remains of a cow's heart attached to his genitals; wires had been attached to the heart and plugged into a wall socket. Ritual murder was discounted after the remains of underground pornographic magazines were found in the boy's room. One of these gave details of a sex toy where a beating heart was used for masturbation purposes. The boy's error was connecting it to the mains and not batteries. An officer on the scene commented, 'This is one of the most gruesome things I have ever seen. I can't believe that there are people who actually enjoy this sort of thing.'

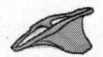

Burglar Paul Mountain, thirty-eight, of Darwen, Lancashire broke into a shed but was arrested after having sex with a teddy bear and leaving his DNA as evidence. Mr Mountain told police that he was coming down from an amphetamine high and felt an 'overwhelming need' for sexual relief. Blackburn Magistrates Court heard that the owner of an allotment found her shed had been broken into and she found the abused teddy bear on the floor. It was passed to police, who discovered semen inside a hole made in the toy. The thief pleaded guilty to burglary with intent to steal. What happened to the bear was not reported.

In a similar incident, a Cincinnati man was arrested in June 2012 and charged with exposing himself and masturbating with a teddy bear. This was his fourth arrest in two years for the same offence.

MAN DIES DURING SEX WITH SCARECROW HE DRESSED IN LIPSTICK AND LONG-HAIRED WIG is not the sort of headline you see every day. The story refers to fifty-eight-year-old shepherd Jose Alberto, who lived in San Jose de Balcarce, Argentina. In April 2015, after neighbours reported a rotting smell coming from his home, police broke in to find his decomposing remains next to a scarecrow that had been dressed as a woman but with a six-inch strap-on dildo fixed to it. Police spokesman Rodulfo Moure said, 'I initially thought there were two bodies but then I realised one was a scarecrow wearing lipstick and a long-haired wig.' Neighbours said that Sr Alberto was known as a loner.

Sharkur Lucas – a mortuary worker in Ghana – told a local TV station that he was unable to get women to go out with him due to his morbid job so, instead, he turned to the next best thing: having sex with the corpses. He also claimed he was told by his superiors that sex with the bodies was part of his training and that, to date, he'd had relations with a hundred bodies. When the interviewer raised the question of mental-health problems, Mr Lucas insisted that he was 'OK.' Since the interview was broadcast in April 2015, the mortuary worker has been sacked by his employers and is being sought by the police, although he apparently remains convinced he did nothing wrong.

There's so much wrong with this sentence: Roman Emperor Nero used to dress young boys in his dead wife's clothes and have sex with them.

THAT'S JUST WRONG!

In 1995 Stephen N. Porco, twenty-eight, was sentenced to six years in prison for a series of car thefts in and around Knoxville, Tennessee. He'd break into the vehicles and steal women's purses – not for their contents but, instead, was using them for what reports called 'sexual gratification'. Porco was said to have had this fetish for at least ten years, during which time he was estimated to have stolen over 500 purses.

A fifty-three-year-old male nurse from Oregon was charged with pandering obscenity when his collection of photographs of corpses came to light. According to the Sheriff's Department, the man had been fired by one hospital for 'spending too much time with cadavers.' After his arrest, the man admitted that he found the photos sexually exciting. He was caught after staff at a photo-developing service found the photos of the dead bodies arranged in various disturbing positions and alerted the police.

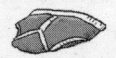

A marathon runner was arrested for covertly filming women competitors urinating during a race. Unrepentant, when the case came to court, he told the judge, 'If the runners are going to do that sort of thing in public, they should expect people to see them.' The court heard that, while filming, the accused was dressed as a giant banana.

IS IT IN YET?

In 2006, armed with shovels, a crowbar and a box of condoms, three men broke into a cemetery in Cassville in south-western Wisconsin, in order to have sex with the body of a twenty-year-old woman who'd been killed the week before in a motorcycle accident. The court heard that one of the trio had been attracted to the pretty nursing assistant after seeing her obituary photo in the local newspaper and had asked the others for help digging up her corpse. They'd used the shovels to reach her grave but were unable to pry open the concrete vault. The men were discovered by a police officer responding to reports of a suspicious vehicle in the cemetery and charged with attempted sexual assault and theft.

At first, a judge dismissed the assault charges, saying Wisconsin law does not criminalise necrophilia. However, an appeals court upheld the decision that assault victims can be dead or alive.

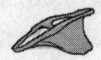

The most famous modern-day necrophiliac was former policeman and civil servant Dennis Nilsen who, in 1983, admitted killing 'fifteen or sixteen' young men in his north London home and then having sex with and masturbating over their dead bodies, even while he cut them up. At his trial, Nilsen claimed that his passion for this behaviour was so intense that he could have continued 'until I was sixty-five.'

THAT'S JUST WRONG!

Three months after the death of his fiancée in a motorcycle accident, twenty-one-year-old Roberto Carlos da Silva of Sorocaba, Brazil dug up her body and had sex with it. He later told the Estado news agency, 'I was desperate and needed her.' The report stated that police were awaiting the results of a psychiatric examination before deciding whether to indict him.

Jeffrey Watkins, twenty-four, was convicted in 1994 of breaking into and committing thefts from five mausoleums at Mt Hope Cemetery in Rochester, New York. At his trial, Watkins confessed he'd often slept with the remains inside coffins, declaring, 'I feel safe with the dead and I can trust them.'

A thirty-five-year-old man was admitted to his local ER suffering from severe abdominal pain and a subsequent X-ray showed multiple small rounded objects in his stomach. Doctors suspected he'd ingested packets filled with illicit drugs for the purpose of smuggling. However, the patient admitted that the objects were actually Barbie-doll heads, swallowed over the course of several days for the purpose of anal autoerotic gratification. He and fellow devotees of this fixation would wait until the doll's head entered their rectums, at which point they'd reach in and get off by suddenly yanking it out by the hair.

IS IT IN YET?

Sixty-two-year-old Reverend Emyr Owen – a Methodist minister from Tywyn, a seaside resort in west Wales – demonstrated the sort of behaviour you wouldn't expect from a man of the cloth: molesting corpses. In 1985 he confessed to mutilating three bodies after they'd been laid out in a chapel of rest. He admitted injecting some of the penises with boiling water after he'd chopped them off, so they'd stand erect. When police raided his home, they found a collection of S&M pornography and three photographs of dismembered penises and scrotums arranged on plates.

The minister served four years in prison but the dismembered penises were never produced in court as evidence. Jurors heard that one had been fed to the seagulls on Tywyn beach, another burned and a third thrown in the sea.

In 1979 a Californian mortuary assistant stole a male corpse from a hearse and drove him into the mountains, where she proceeded to abuse the body (well, as much as she could, considering his state). She was traced and arrested but the only things she could be charged with were stealing a hearse and interfering with a burial, for which she received a fine of $200 and a week in jail.

THAT'S JUST WRONG!

German-born Carl Tanzler was a radiographer at the United States Marine Hospital in Key West, Florida who developed a sexual obsession for a young Cuban-American TB patient, Elena Milagro de Hoyos, that continued well after her death from the disease in 1931.

Removing her body from its tomb, he lived with the corpse at his home, using copious amounts of perfume to mask the smell. In October 1940, after hearing a series of rumours, Elena's sister, Florinda, confronted Tanzler at his house and discovered the disinterred body and the full extent of his obsession. He'd replaced decomposing skin with plaster of Paris, fitted glass eyes and filled her abdominal cavity with rags to maintain the body's shape. He'd also inserted a paper tube in the corpse's vagina so that he could have intercourse with it.

Tanzler stood trial on the charge of 'wantonly and maliciously destroying a grave and removing a body without authorization' but the case had to be dropped, since the statute of limitations had expired and Tanzler moved away from the area.

The case was a sensation among the public, who were generally sympathetic to Tanzler, who was just viewed as an 'eccentric romantic'.

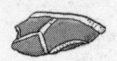

In 1849 Parisian police sergeant François Bertrand was arrested after being discovered digging up corpses from the city's Père Lachaise and Montparnasse cemeteries in order to have sex with them. He also liked biting the corpses

IS IT IN YET?

and many were found with teeth marks over them. He was convicted of fifteen counts but served just one year in prison.

When Thai police arrested thirty-five-year-old Buddhist monk Samai Parnthong for having sex with the corpse of a forty-year-old woman, they were unable to find a law against necrophilia. Instead, they charged him with criminal damage to a coffin.

Thirty-seven-year-old Donald Baker of Santa Barbara was a peeping Tom with a difference. In August 1987 he was arrested by park rangers in the Montana de Oro State Park in California after being seen hiding in a cesspit under the park's primitive female toilets. He was spotted through a crack in the wall by a man waiting for his wife and, when the rangers arrived, they found Baker sitting on a crate wearing protecting clothing and rubber gloves, waist deep in waste. He was hauled out, hosed down and taken to the nearby San Luis Obispo County Jail.

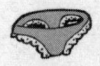

Karl Watkins appeared at Hereford Crown Court in February 1993 charged with five counts of outraging public decency. He'd been caught with his trousers round his ankles, trying to have sex with the pavement. Even an eighteen-month prison sentence wasn't enough to dissuade him; two years later Watkins appeared in court again for attempting to have sex in public with some black plastic bin bags. He revealed a nine-year fetish with the plastic sacks and admitted that his ultimate sexual fantasy was to be in the back of dustcart when the bin bags were crushed. Watkins was put on three years' probation and ordered to seek psychiatric help.

In a similar case, Ross Watt, twenty-eight, was arrested in Edinburgh after he was found by police one morning having sex with a shoe in the street. Sheriff Richard Scott told Watt, 'If you have to do things like this, then do them in private.'

An anonymous twenty-nine-year-old man from North Carolina was arrested in 1998, 2003 and 2007 for the same crime: theft to satisfy his bizarre sexual fetish. He stole soiled baby nappies from bins. He told police that he liked to wear the nappies for a sexual thrill and that the fact they were dirty gave him a little extra stimulation. He was actually caught after he reached into a car and attempted to remove a soiled nappy. He was put on probation for three years.

IS IT IN YET?

If you thought that flavoured and even luminous condoms were 'out there', think again. They're positively passé when you consider that you can now buy condoms shaped like dinosaurs, bananas and the devil – or, for Easter, condoms ribbed to resemble a crown of thorns. For those who want to impress their partner, there are condoms printed with a ruler (presumably one that takes into account stretching) and, for the style conscious, there are condoms that resemble a tuxedo or a Louis Vuitton bag. And if the only thing big about you is your ego, you can even have condoms printed with your face and name.

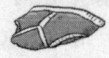

A&E staff are used to patients turning up with foreign objects embedded in their rectums (usually 'completely by accident'). However, one of the oddest cases involved a concrete enema. The victim explained that his friend had poured a mixture of cement and sand into his rectum via a funnel but they'd left it too long and the mixture had hardened into concrete. Fortunately, surgeons managed to remove it during a lengthy operation, leaving the patient with a unique and very personal souvenir of their exploits – a perfect concrete cast of his rectum.

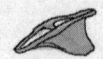

'Pumping away' took on a new meaning for a thirteen-year-old Thai boy Charnchai Puanmuangpak. According to a report in *The Japan Times* in April 1997, the boy was heavily

THAT'S JUST WRONG!

into a craze among young men of inserting a bicycle pump into their rectums so that the sudden rush of air creates a momentary high. In order to increase his pleasure, Charnchai went a step too far. He and some friends went to a petrol station, where he inserted an airline deep into his rectum. Within moments of him placing a coin into the slot to start the air, he exploded. A spokesman for the Maharat Nakhon Ratchasima Hospital later commented, 'When that quantity of air interacted with the gas in his system, it was like an atom bomb went off. We still haven't located all of him.'

Australian William J. Chidley (1860–1916) was a self-styled social reformer with many unconventional views. The most extreme was his theory that it was wrong to have an erect penis during sex. He claimed this was unnatural and produced shocks to both men and women. Instead, he promoted what he called the 'crowbar method', whereby a flaccid penis is inserted into the woman, drawn in by a vacuum in the vagina (he stated that this vacuum would only occur in the spring). Preaching these views in public, Chidley was charged with offensive behaviour, pronounced insane and sent to a Sydney asylum, where he died.

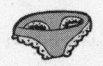

Poet Lord Byron and Lady Caroline Lamb expressed their true love for one another by exchanging locks of their pubic hair.

IS IT IN YET?

An Edinburgh man who was caught having sex with a traffic cone claimed that he was just performing a piece of 'fringe street theatre.' Given that it was the time of the Edinburgh Festival, the judge believed his excuse and declined to pass sentence, providing the act was never repeated again.

In April 2008 Daniel French, twenty-four, broke into the locked Leicester Square Gardens in central London and was seen by police making 'sexual motions' with metal railings. Westminster Magistrates Court was told that he said words to the effect of, 'I'm going to have sex with that fence.' French, of Stevenage, Hertfordshire, admitted being drunk and disorderly after a night out in the West End but angrily denied making romantic overtures towards the fence. He was sentenced to serve the time he had already spent in custody since his arrest — meaning he was allowed to walk free from court.

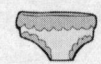

Objectophiles is the name given to those people who develop significant relationships with inanimate objects. One of the most famous is Erika LaBrie — an American who married the Eiffel Tower in a commitment ceremony in 2007 — changing her name afterwards to Erika La Tour Eiffel. Erika first encountered the monument in 2004 and said she felt an immediate attraction, telling ABC News that she and others like her 'feel an innate connection to objects.

THAT'S JUST WRONG!

It comes perfectly normal to us to connect on various levels, emotional, spiritual and also physical for some.'

Erika is a former archery world champion and continues to compete at an international level, claiming that her relationship with Lance – her competition bow – helped her to become a world-class archer.

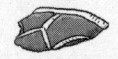

SAYINGS ABOUT SEX

Not everyone waxes lyrically about the celebration, gratification and satisfaction of sex. For example, Lord Chesterfield once said, 'The position is undignified, the pleasure momentary and the consequences utterly damnable.' Many other notable people agree…

Sex is the biggest nothing of all time.
Andy Warhol

All this fuss about sleeping together. For physical pleasure, I'd sooner go to my dentist any day.
Evelyn Waugh

IS IT IN YET?

I'm at the age where food has taken the place of sex in my life. In fact, I've just had a mirror put over my kitchen table.
Rodney Dangerfield

The next time you feel desire coming on, don't give way to it. If you have the chance, just wash your parts in cold water and cool them down.
Lord Baden-Powell (advice to boy scouts)

Sex is a bad thing because it rumples the clothes.
Jacqueline Kennedy Onassis

Sex at age ninety is like trying to shoot pool with a rope.
George Burns

I know [sex] makes people happy but, to me, it's just like having a cup of tea.
Cynthia Payne

SAYINGS ABOUT SEX

I would rather have a cup of tea than sex.
Boy George

Don't knock masturbation. It's sex with someone I love.
Woody Allen

It's been so long since I've had sex, I've forgotten who ties up whom.
Joan Rivers

Guns don't kill people; husbands that come home early kill people.
Don Rose

I am just as unsatisfied the morning after as I am the night before.
Sarah Bernhardt

Sex is interesting but it's not totally important.
Charles Bukowski

IS IT IN YET?

Sexual intercourse is like having someone else blow your nose.
Philip Larkin

I know nothing about sex because I was always married.
Zsa Zsa Gabor

The big difference between sex for money and sex for free is that sex for money usually costs a lot less.
Brendan Behan

I remember the first time I had sex. I kept the receipt.
Groucho Marx

Sex is simple once you realise it's just like riding a bicycle. In both cases, the hardest part is learning not to fall off.
Jim Riffe

Masturbation is the thinking man's television.
Christopher Hampton

SAYINGS ABOUT SEX

The only reason I feel guilty about masturbation is because I do it so badly.
David Steinberg

A man marries to have a home but also because he doesn't want to be bothered with sex and all that sort of thing.
W. Somerset Maugham

Having sex is like playing bridge. If you don't have a good partner, you'd better have a good hand.
Woody Allen

Excessive wealth and excessive perversion go hand in hand.
Monique van Vooren

There is no unhappier creature on earth than a fetishist who yearns for a woman's shoes and has to embrace the whole woman.
Karl Kraus

IS IT IN YET?

What's the three words you never want to hear while making love? 'Honey, I'm home!'
Ken Hammond

My love life is terrible. The last time I was inside a woman was when I visited the Statue of Liberty.
Woody Allen

There is nothing wrong with going to bed with someone of your own sex. People should be very free with sex. They should draw the line at goats.
Elton John

Skiing is better than sex, actually, because, for me, a good round of sex might be seven minutes. Skiing you can do for seven hours.
Spalding Gray